CONNECTED FOR HEALTH

CONNECTED FOR HEALTH

Using Electronic Health Records to Transform Care Delivery

Louise L. Liang, Editor

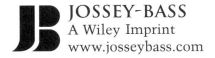
JOSSEY-BASS
A Wiley Imprint
www.josseybass.com

Published by Jossey-Bass
A Wiley Imprint
989 Market Street, San Francisco, CA 94103-1741—www.josseybass.com

Jossey-Bass books and products are available through most bookstores. To contact Jossey-Bass directly call our Customer Care Department within the U.S. at 800-956-7739, outside the U.S. at 317-572-3986, or fax 317-572-4002.

Jossey-Bass also publishes its books in a variety of electronic formats. Some content that appears in print may not be available in electronic books.

Library of Congress Cataloging-in-Publication Data

Cataloging-in-publication data has been applied for.
ISBN: 978-0-4706-3937-5

Printed in the United States of America
FIRST EDITION
HB Printing   10 9 8 7 6 5 4 3 2

CONTENTS

To my husband, Richard, and my children, Margot and Ethan,
whose support and understanding throughout my career ensured
that I was ready for the opportunity of a lifetime

"Do not go where the path may lead, go instead where there is no path and leave a trail."

—Ralph Waldo Emerson

ACKNOWLEDGMENTS

In any major undertaking, there are many people without whom there would be no story, certainly not with a happy ending. KP HealthConnect was no exception. Special thanks go to George Halvorson, CEO, Kaiser Foundation Health Plan and Kaiser Foundation Hospitals, for his vision and unwavering support. Thanks to the Kaiser Foundation Health Plan, Kaiser Foundation Hospitals' board of directors for their farsightedness and confidence in our ability. Thanks to the national leadership team, regional presidents, Permanente executive medical directors, and labor partners for their leadership and commitment. Thanks to Andy Wiesenthal, the Permanente Federation executive sponsor of KP HealthConnect, for his expertise, his dedication, and his support. Thanks to the KP HealthConnect national project team led by Bruce Turkstra, Donna Deckard, Pam Hudson, and Robert Goldstein for their expertise, perseverance, and good humor in the face of unparalleled challenges. Thanks to the hundreds of regional and national staff whose work was dedicated to implementing or leveraging KP HealthConnect to make care and operations better. Thanks to Judy Faulkner, CEO, and Carl Dvorak, COO, of Epic Systems, and the hundreds of Epic staff for understanding and translating what we needed. Thanks to Jason Girzadas, Lynne Sterrett, and Kevin McCarter, Deloitte Consulting, whose counsel and staff helped us over many rough spots. Thanks to Don Berwick, CEO, and Maureen Bisognano, COO, Institute for Healthcare Improvement, for sharing our vision for health care in the future and working with us to create it.

When word got out that we were writing a book about KP HealthConnect, many people at Kaiser Permanente came forward to offer their stories. Stories from information technology professionals who had worked on previous projects and told me that KP HealthConnect was the best project they ever worked on. Stories that recall the complex selection process and preparation. Stories that describe the stressful implementations of multiple software applications. And finally, stories about how KP HealthConnect has affected our work, our patients, and the quality of care we provide.

Unfortunately we could not include all these wonderful stories. We have chosen those that capture the special nature of this work and represent similar stories, all key to our success. We thank the thousands of individuals throughout Kaiser Permanente who are not named here but without whom KP HealthConnect would not have been possible. This includes virtually all of the staff and physicians in Kaiser Permanente, whose daily work has been irrevocably changed.

Without KP HealthConnect, there would be no story. And without a dedicated support team and committed contributing authors, there would be no book. Thanks to each and every author—dozens who wrote or contributed to the various chapters so that the full richness of the implementation and leverage of KP HealthConnect could be shared.

Thanks to my overall book editor and organizer, Jon Stewart, director, Special Projects, Kaiser Foundation Health Plan, without whose experience and diligence this book would not have seen print. Thanks, too, to the dedicated team that helped with the myriad tasks of scheduling, editing, revising, fact-checking, layout, sense making, and prodding: Ann Bundy, Mike Lassiter, and Laura Tollen for excellent project management and editing assistance; Keith Paulsen, Ravi Poorsina, and Samantha Quattrone for valuable advice and counsel; and Karen Borst-Rothe for copyediting. Thanks to our internal reviewers, Andy Wiesenthal, MD, associate executive director, Permanente Federation, and Murray Ross, vice president and director, KP Institute of Health Policy, who helped ensure that this book captures the KP HealthConnect story accurately and clearly for our readers. Thanks to our sponsors, Diane Gage-Lofgren, senior vice president, Brand Strategy, Communications, and Public Relations, Kaiser Foundation Health Plan, and John Nelson, vice president, Issues and Brand Management, for providing the resources and staff that supported this book. Thanks, finally, to Andy Pasternack, our editor at Jossey-Bass, for his encouragement and support in bringing our story to print.

THE EDITOR

Louise L. Liang, MD, serves as an executive consultant to Kaiser Foundation Health Plan and speaks, writes, and consults on a broad set of health care issues including electronic information systems, quality, safety, service, and practice redesign. From 2002 to 2009, she served as senior vice president, Quality and Clinical Systems Support, Kaiser Foundation Health Plan and Kaiser Foundation Hospitals, Inc. Working with leaders throughout Kaiser Permanente, she oversaw the national quality agenda to ensure that members received excellent care and service. She led the development and implementation of Kaiser Permanente HealthConnect, a $4 billion-plus organization-wide electronic health record and administrative system to support continuity and quality of care as well as efficient business functions.

From 2000 to 2002, Dr. Liang served as chair, Board of Directors, Institute for Healthcare Improvement. From 1997 to 2001, she served as the chief operating officer and medical director of Group Health Cooperative in Seattle, providing health care services and health insurance to 600,000 people in Washington and northern Idaho. She oversaw delivery system operations, health plan medical policy, and clinical quality. Dr. Liang was also the founding CEO and president of Group Health Permanente, a professional corporation of more than a thousand health professionals that contracts with Group Health Cooperative to provide and manage medical services. From 1992 to 1997, she was chief operating officer for the Straub Clinic and Hospital, a private, multispecialty health care system in Honolulu. Prior to that, Dr. Liang was associate medical director at the Harvard Community Health Plan in Boston, where she was responsible for health center operations.

Previously, Dr. Liang served as the division director, New England Region, Public Health Service; program director, National Childhood Immunization Initiative, Office of the Assistant Secretary of Health; special assistant to the secretary, Department of Health and Human Services; White House fellow; and chief of pediatrics at the Henry Ford Hospital, Fairlane Center. In addition, she served on the Massachusetts Board of Registration of Medicine.

Dr. Liang received her MD from Georgetown University School of Medicine and trained as a pediatrician at the Boston Floating Hospital/Tufts University, New England Medical Center. She served as assistant pediatrician at the Massachusetts General Hospital and clinical instructor at the Harvard Medical School from 1983 through 1992. She is board certified by the American Board of Pediatrics and the American Board of Medical Management.

Dr. Liang served on the Malcolm Baldrige National Quality Award panel of judges during 1998 and 1999, on the Leadership Council of the American Association of Health Plans during 2000 and 2001, and on various other boards and committees.

FOREWORD

By Donald M. Berwick, MD

Health care has a serious case of techno-envy, at least when it comes to information systems. That's a paradox, since it's hard to think of any other industry—aerospace, maybe—more deeply invested in the latest-and-greatest gizmos. No sooner does a new imaging machine or fiber-optic surgery tool hit the market than the doctors line up at both the exhibit hall booth and the hospital budgeting office to get it into the picture, their requests fueled by dramatic claims of benefit to patients and contributions to efficiency. "Not being modern" ranks high among the generators of guilt among both clinicians and health care executives. Heaven forbid that we're behind the times!

So it's curious that health care has found itself so far behind the times in the forms of technology perhaps most powerfully related to its performance, or shortcomings thereof: the technologies that help us manage knowledge, communication, and information: "IT." Most doctors order their novels online but write prescriptions with pen and paper. Most nurses watch their pizza joint clerk enter their orders on a touch screen but hand-write patients' vital signs hundreds of times a day in thick, unreadable paper records. To call health care's information management for the most part "twentieth century" is as wrong as calling it "twenty-first century"; it's nineteenth century.

Donald M. Berwick, MD, MPP, is president and CEO of the Institute for Healthcare Improvement.

For three decades or more, we've all known how costly that gap is. The first Institute of Medicine (IOM) Committee I ever sat on was called "The Committee on the Future of the Patient Record." That was in 1989, and its hard-hitting report lamented twenty years of failure to adopt widely the computerized patient record. It called for immediate action.

We're still waiting, sort of. I write "sort of" because there is also a positive side of the story: enormous advances, still accelerating, in tools and techniques for better and better management of the terabyte-sized reservoir of clinical and scientific knowledge that we should bring to the service of patients; speedier, more reliable, and secure communication among clinicians and between clinicians and patients; and far more useable, accurate, and intelligent ways to store and retrieve information about individual patients themselves.

Better, also, are the ways in which patients, families, and communities can get access to previously locked-up knowledge about the diseases that afflict them, the risks that threaten them, and the treatments that can help them. With respect to their health and health care, countless laypeople have now made the shift from benighted to savvy to expert, and the smart doctor today asks patients to report what they have found on the Web that the doctor doesn't know yet. Pioneering health care organizations and systems, such as the Veterans Health Administration and the Indian Health Service, and our foremost multispecialty group practice systems, such as Mayo Clinic, Geisinger Health System, Cleveland Clinic, and Kaiser Permanente, have developed and adopted clinical and managerial information systems that would do NASA proud. The National Library of Medicine is, by any measure, a jewel in the crown of federal function and is widely admired for its modernity. Information technology innovators are hard at work, and their wares have increasing glitz and functionality. The Healthcare Information Management and Systems Society annual conference has become one of the largest in the whole health care industry.

And, let it not go unnoticed that, in the flurry of U.S. government responses to the financial meltdown of 2008–2009, the federal "stimulus package" included $19 billion for the Department of Health and Human Services to invest in helping American health care providers adopt information technologies to support patient care.

But it is not yet time for celebration; not even close. If the 1989 IOM Committee on the Future of the Patient Record were empanelled today, it could just about Xerox its 1990 report and call it a day. The numbers tell a good part of the story: as of 2009, only 9 percent of America's hospitals were using even a basic form of electronic medical records (Jha and others, 2009) and, as of 2008, only 13 percent of America's practicing doctors were doing so (DesRoches, 2008). And, looking deeper, an even smaller fraction of those that had "computerization" has anything close to the functionality that you meet every day in every Wal-Mart.

Why the gap? It's not as if we cannot imagine the benefits that twenty-first-century information management could bring both to patients and to those who serve them; any eighty-year-old probably could imagine that today, between sessions on Google, Facebook, and Guitar Hero. And it's not as if we don't have some promising prototypes. I have practiced pediatrics in both the now-departed HMO, the Harvard Community Health Plan, and the Indian Health Service in Alaska, and in both I used computer records, electronic consultations, and computer decision supports.

It's not as if the need for modernization hasn't increased—a lot—since the fretful 1989 IOM Committee met. Indeed, the case for change took a giant step forward in 2001, from rhetoric to evidence, in the form of another IOM report, *Crossing the Quality Chasm* (Institute of Medicine, 2001), the most important single chartering document for health care redesign and improvement in my entire career.

Famously, and of crucial importance, the *Chasm* report gave us "aims for improvement"—six, to be specific: "Safety, Effectiveness, Patient-Centeredness, Timeliness, Efficiency, and Equity." For me, and for many of my colleagues, that list is now canonical—it guides our efforts every day. And modernizing the way our industry handles knowledge, communication, and patient information is a key to progress in every single one of those dimensions—not sufficient by any stretch, but almost certainly necessary. For example,

- *Safer* care can benefit from the automation of knowledge, surveillance, alarms, and signaling that can outdo the best human mind any day of the week. It can alert the doctor who prescribed an incompatible medication, help a nurse to know when trouble is afoot, render confusing information orderly and illegible information readable. It can speed awareness of a hazard from the first place it is noticed to every place and person that needs to know. It can bridge across sites of care, unifying time and space, and thereby make handoffs and coordination more secure.
- More *effective* care can come from new forms of access to copious knowledge. One source tells me that over 40,000 clinical trials are under way in the world at any one time now. A doctor who read one of those a day would be a century behind in her reading by year's end. Only a post-Google world can solve that problem. Modern diagnostic and treatment algorithms can now be made automatic—if the doctor chooses—freeing the clinician's mind from tasks of memory far beyond reasonable to ask them to perform. Databases, carefully managed and nurtured, can reveal patterns of overuse, underuse, error, and hazard that, in a more primitive information system, simply cannot be known because they cannot be seen.
- *Patient-centered* care in this millennium has a whole new set of demands and opportunities. People can, with proper support, take a far larger role in ensuring their own health and participating in their own care; those with chronic illness can find continuity and memory among the sites and clinicians who care for them, instead of feeling lost and confused; communication between clinicians and patients can be far easier and multimodal, making the former mainstay of care—the "visit"— only one among the ways to get and give help, and not often the best one, at that;

and patients can communicate with each other, to share common experiences and lessons learned.

- *Timeliness* is a direct benefit of modernization, as the flow of electrons at light speed replaces the automobile and shoe leather as the common way to move what we need and need to know. For a simple question and answer, e-mail beats a visit almost every single time. Information technology gives us a chance to pattern flows and predict demand and supply to erase waits and reduce inventories through the prompt and proper use of knowledge.
- *Efficiency* is a close relative to much of the above, since defects in safety, effectiveness, timeliness, and patient-centered care all amount to forms of waste as well as poor experiences. But modern IT goes even further in helping discover where value resides and doesn't. It can allow the supply chain to flow with far less viscosity, and it can identify innovations and spread the news.
- *Equity*, the most elusive of the IOM six aims, stands to gain as well if (and yes, yes, it is a big "if") we can close the "Digital Divide." After all, the "send" button doesn't know your race or your wealth, and good computer patient records will allow us to spot and name instances where our actions don't match our words when it comes to disadvantaged populations. Even language barriers may begin to fall as twenty-first-century word processing and communication systems get better at managing translation.

The promise of modern information technology in health care is as prodigious as the gap in adopting it is wide.

But here comes Kaiser Permanente's KP HealthConnect. I first became aware of it when Kaiser Permanente leaders asked the Institute for Healthcare Improvement to help with KP HealthConnect, especially with respect to its intended function: to transform health care. Like the foresighted leaders they are, George Halvorson, Louise Liang, and their colleagues knew, absolutely, that the technology of KP HealthConnect, as necessary as it would be, would be only part of the story. Without clear incorporation into the actual processes of care, and without the re-engineering of those processes, and without the changes in norms, capabilities, and culture to allow those new systems to take root, KP HealthConnect would become what far too many other health care organizations had already discovered in their own modernization journeys: the computerization of a defective *status quo*. Kaiser Permanente was not after a modern *information* system; they were after a modern *health care* system. Halvorson called building KP HealthConnect "laying tracks," but he and I both knew that, in the end, it would be the trains, not the tracks, that mattered more.

Appropriately, the shared work of IHI and the Kaiser Permanente team used a framework—the 21st Century Care Innovation Project—much broader than simply modernizing information management. KP HealthConnect found its leverage in a reconceptualization of care itself, and through refreshed thinking about how knowledge helps patients. I found the most exciting idea in the thrilling and portentous rubric "Home as the hub" from the vision Kaiser Permanente had developed for health care in the future. In these four words, Kaiser Permanente recentered the tasks of care, healing, and prevention exactly where they belong—in the normal, daily lives of people, well and ill alike, and drawing on all the resources that they and we can bring to bear to help them thrive. "Home as the hub" liberates the pursuit of health—our real aim—from the pursuit of health care, which is merely a tool for achieving that aim. And with wise redesign concepts in play, KP HealthConnect could become the most helpful single asset for realizing that redesign—not technology for its own sake, but technology for health's sake.

I wasn't sure they could pull it off. The enormous scale of the process changes required to care differently for almost nine million people was paired with the enormous changes in beliefs and habits of the workforce that would be required to make the new care real. KP HealthConnect was no "plug and play" device; it was one edge of a wholesale reconsideration of health care itself that would cut deeply into long-cherished norms and expectations. This was a change that demanded courage, teamwork, and trust in nearly unprecedented measure.

But they did it. Today, Kaiser Permanente's leaders would be the first to acknowledge that even more changes lie ahead, and that their journey into modernized care with modernized information technology is still young. Nonetheless, drawing on the almost unfair advantage of their nature as a truly integrated care system, using the leverage of consolidated budgets and long-sighted investment, and harnessing the creativity of an entire workforce right down to their valued front-line teams, Kaiser Permanente has shown truly what "modern" can mean when twenty-first-century information becomes the servant it can be to twenty-first-century patients and families. When it comes to IT, Kaiser Permanente need envy no longer; it's time now for others to both envy and emulate them.

As American health care continues to struggle with challenges of quality, public satisfaction, and cost, there are lessons for all parts of our health care system. Those who provide and insure health care; those who use and pay for health care; and finally those who define the framework for the U.S. health care system through policy, regulation, and funding will learn what is possible when a health care system is allowed to innovate and improve in a setting with appropriate financial and professional incentives. The story of KP HealthConnect and its impact on the delivery of safe, effective care is dramatic and compelling—hopefully, a glimpse of the future.

INTRODUCTION

By Louise L. Liang, MD

In early 2010, Kaiser Permanente completed the implementation of KP Health-Connect, the largest nongovernmental electronic health record (EHR) in the world. This book is about how it changed our organization and the health care we provide our members. We hope that it will inform leaders and stakeholders who are committed to improving health care and health for patients and families, who deserve safer, more effective health care in more convenient, customized ways.

Our experience, related throughout this book, demonstrates that the availability of comprehensive health information to all care providers, as well as to patients, provides the foundation for a fundamental rethinking of the delivery of health care—who provides care, how care is provided, and what care outcomes are achievable. Although we recognize that the comprehensive and integrated Kaiser Permanente health care system, with its aligned financial incentives for quality, gave us a special opportunity to redesign care, there are lessons here for all stakeholders in American health care: policy makers, regulators, those who pay for and receive health care, and those who deliver health care.

The Long Journey to KP HealthConnect

The developmental pathway to KP HealthConnect began in the early 1960s when Kaiser Permanente's founding physician, Sidney Garfield, MD, asked his colleague,

Morris Collen, MD, director of Kaiser Permanente's first medical research center, to attend a national congress on medical electronics. Collen, who has a degree in electrical engineering, returned convinced that there were ways to use computers to improve health care. With support from Garfield, Collen received a grant from the U.S. Public Health Service in 1962 to study the computerized automation of multiphasic health testing, a program he had led since the early 1950s. As a result of this project, Kaiser Permanente patients were among the first in the world to see internists armed with computer printouts of pertinent medical data.

Other federal grants to Kaiser Permanente for the computerization of medical information, including clinical, pharmaceutical, and lab data, followed during the 1960s and 1970s. By 1979 the automated multiphasic testing program had accumulated fifteen years of longitudinal health data from a half million patient examinations. The data provided solid evidence of reduced morbidity, mortality, and disability among older members who had been through the automated multiphasic testing process as well as data for more than 150 additional clinical research publications.

By the late 1980s and throughout the 1990s, almost every one of Kaiser Permanente's regional operating units across the United States—in Hawaii, northern and southern California, the Northwest, Colorado, Ohio, the mid-Atlantic states, and Georgia—was working on the development or implementation of some form of a localized health IT system, including patient records. While advanced for the health care industry, each of these separate efforts was confined to ambulatory care, not hospital care, and they could not support the full integration and coordination of care across all medical specialties and care settings, much less include patient access to the medical record. Different EHR structures and software programs had led to many different IT applications, processes, and standards, each customized to regional needs and preferences but very little that was developed in one area could benefit others— even when the separate regions wanted to share their successes.

Forging a Common EHR Solution—and a Unified Organization

As the 1990s ended, a sea-change decision by Kaiser Permanente's senior leadership led the organization in a new direction—the development of a single, comprehensive electronic health record (EHR) that would serve all of Kaiser Permanente, from Hawaii to Washington, D.C.

The work since then has offered a myriad of challenges, not the least of which was the requirement for complex interfaces with each region's multiple legacy systems. In the clinical area alone, there were more than 250 legacy systems that had to be interfaced to the new EHR, at least until the new system was completely implemented. Just the task of selecting a vendor for the new system—a system that had to satisfy more than 14,000 physicians, 45,000 nurses, and thousands of other clinicians and staff—required months of study and compromises on everyone's part.

In the process of all this, we also had to confront the many barriers, both cultural and operational, to working efficiently as a single organization—not something Kaiser Permanente, as a collection of regional operations, was accustomed to doing. But by having to come together around something as central and transformative as a common EHR, we learned how to come together as a single, national organization while still allowing and encouraging regional innovation and adaptation of program-wide initiatives, as needed.

What follows is the story of how market forces; human nature; and especially the realization that the patient, not the medical professional, needs to be at the center of any real reform of health care delivery led to the development of KP HealthConnect. This is a classic story of strategic direction and change management, of aspirations and day-to-day reality, of calculated risk-taking and experienced judgment.

After all, this was not merely a big IT project. It was putting down the infrastructure for redefining and transforming health care.

Overview of Contents

In planning this book, we determined early on that it was important that it reflect the many perspectives and experiences of Kaiser Permanente physicians and staff who helped implement KP HealthConnect and whose work has been affected by it. Consequently, several of the chapters have been written by multiple authors, and most chapters include short contributions, or sidebars, by additional authors: physician leaders, health plan and hospital leaders, nurses, pharmacists, quality and safety experts, labor leaders, and health care researchers.

In organizing the content, we have grouped the twelve chapters into four sections that address the overall themes of this book: strategic leadership, KP HealthConnect implementation, harvesting value from KP HealthConnect, and future opportunities for computerized health care.

Section One, "Setting the Course," describes the organizational context that led to the strategic decision to implement a single electronic health record to leverage Kaiser Permanente's already formidable clinical assets. Chapter One discusses the driving forces and strategic rationale for the implementation of KP HealthConnect. It reviews how the project leadership led development of an organization-wide vision for what health care, enabled by an EHR, could and should look like fifteen years out, and how that vision has continued to guide the implementation and value realization of KP HealthConnect.

Section Two, "Laying the Tracks," outlines the collaborative approach to the implementation of KP HealthConnect and how it positioned the organization for the achievement of value. The first challenge, described in Chapter Two, involved the development of a national software platform and shared clinical tools that balanced the standardization required for efficient system operation, data collection and processing, and performance improvement, and the customization required for varying regional regulations, operational priorities, and legacy systems. There was no precedent for a project of this size or complexity. A new structure, approaches, and culture were developed through an approach named the "collaborative build" to engage the eight Kaiser Permanente regions and all key stakeholders in ensuring a successful project, as well as new ways for Kaiser Permanente to move forward as an aligned organization in other undertakings. Chapter Three addresses the key roles that three different types of physician leaders played in ensuring that success—operational leaders, opinion leaders, and technically adept physicians.

Chapter Four reviews the roles of another key stakeholder group, nursing leaders, in developing and implementing KP HealthConnect, especially in the inpatient (hospital) setting. A case study at the end of this section describing one region's experience implementing KP HealthConnect helps illustrate how all of these areas came together.

Section Three, "Harvesting Value," describes how Kaiser Permanente prepared for—and is now realizing—improvements and innovations supported by KP HealthConnect in clinical quality, patient safety, patient access and engagement, care delivery, operations, and clinical research.

Chapter Five provides the conceptual framework for how Kaiser Permanente approached the goals of value realization while reassessing and realigning the organization's quality agenda and infrastructure to take full advantage of KP HealthConnect.

Chapter Six reviews the ways in which the availability of the EHR has enhanced and opened new and innovative approaches in the all-important arena of population-based care management involving both primary care and specialty groups.

Chapter Seven discusses a multiregion quality improvement initiative called the 21st Century Care Innovation Project, which employed more than a dozen clinical teams in investigating ways in which KP HealthConnect could optimize the delivery of quality care while helping alleviate the growing burdens on primary care providers. The chapter includes first-person accounts by three physician leaders who participated in the initiative, each discussing how the EHR has improved the care they deliver and restructured the practice lives of primary care physicians.

Chapter Eight looks at how KP HealthConnect has been configured to enable vastly improved patient engagement in their own health care by giving Kaiser Permanente members a highly secure, Web-based portal into their medical records, known as My Health Manager. Using this personal health record, patients can access most parts of their medical records, including lab results, medical visit summaries, immunization records, and medical histories; communicate online with their physicians; book appointments, and much more (see "Kaiser Permanente HealthConnect: A Primer," following this introduction). The impact of My Health Manager on patients, families, and clinicians has been overwhelmingly positive, as demonstrated by rapidly rising usage rates.

Chapter Nine looks at how KP HealthConnect has automated and enhanced Kaiser Permanente's approaches to patient safety, demonstrated through a number of innovative programs and case studies.

The final chapter in this section, Chapter Ten, reviews the ways in which EHRs generally and KP HealthConnect in particular are helping to develop new medical knowledge as our clinical and health services research colleagues comb through ever larger and more sophisticated databases of clinical information.

Finally, **Section Four,** "Future Directions," describes further opportunities to harness both aggregate and individual health information to improve individual patients, population, and organization-wide outcomes.

Chapter Eleven describes the Archimedes Model, developed by David Eddy, the chapter author, under the sponsorship of Kaiser Permanente. Archimedes is a computer-based mathematical model of human physiology, major diseases, health behaviors, medical interventions, and health care systems. Linked to data from KP HealthConnect, it is providing tools and analyses to help determine the most effective and efficient approaches to care for both patient populations and individual patients—a glimpse of truly customized medicine.

In the closing chapter, Kaiser Foundation Health Plan Chairman and CEO George Halvorson looks at how health information technology can continue to transform the health care delivery system to provide high-quality, affordable care for all Americans. The old path, says Halvorson, has led us to a dead end, but a new path beckons.

KAISER PERMANENTE HEALTHCONNECT: A PRIMER

K aiser Permanente HealthConnect is recognized as the world's largest privately funded electronic health record (EHR). It is a comprehensive health information system that securely connects member records across both ambulatory and inpatient settings; integrates billing, scheduling, and registration; and provides members with access to personal health records on the organization's Web-based member interface, kp.org.

Functionalities

KP HealthConnect, based primarily on software from Epic Systems, of Verona, Wisconsin, seamlessly integrates the following suite of applications:

- *A personal health record,* My Health Manager, available to Kaiser Permanente members beginning in late 2005 on kp.org, now regarded as the world's most broadly and actively used personal health record.
- *Outpatient practice management,* first deployed in late 2003, including billing, registration, and check-in/scheduling. It is now used in all 431 Kaiser Permanente medical office buildings to coordinate outpatient practice management needs.
- *Outpatient clinicals,* including computerized physician order entry (CPOE) and clinical documentation, first deployed in early 2004, completed in early 2008, and

since expanded with new Epic modules to support oncology, home health, radiology, and kiosk check-in.

- *Inpatient billing*, first deployed in late 2004 and now used in all hospitals to coordinate revenue cycle functions.
- *Inpatient pharmacy*, first deployed in late 2004, and used in all hospital pharmacies.
- *Inpatient administrative systems*, including admissions/discharge/transfer (ADT) and emergency department tracker, first deployed in mid-2005 and used in all hospitals to manage census and scheduling needs.
- *Inpatient clinicals*, including bedside clinical documentation, CPOE, emergency department, and operating rooms, first deployed in mid-2006 and since expanded with new modules to support anesthesia and oncology. This is the largest private hospital deployment in the country, including all thirty-five Kaiser Permanente hospitals by the first quarter of 2010.
- *Non-Epic Systems applications* including those provided by IBM, Vignette, Right Fax, Ingenix, and PerSe/Relay Health.
- *Pre-existing applications* that interface with KP HealthConnect including outpatient pharmacy systems, inpatient and outpatient laboratory systems, and radiology systems. In smaller Kaiser Permanente regions, there are major interfaces to approximately ten ancillary systems; in the largest regions, including northern and southern California, the number of interfaces climbs to fifty or more.

KP HealthConnect Users

KP HealthConnect had 82,000 internal active users—Kaiser Permanente employees, clinicians, or physicians with authorized access to one or more applications within KP HealthConnect—by the end of 2007, with many more joining since then. By 2010, the system was averaging about 80,000 concurrent users on any given day. In addition, more than 5,600 affiliated non-Permanente providers in Kaiser Permanente's Mid-Atlantic, Colorado, and Georgia regions who see Kaiser Permanente members are authorized to securely view patient information through a Web portal.

In addition to clinicians and employees, Kaiser Permanente members are able to access portions of their KP HealthConnect records online through their PHR, My Health Manager, which was fully deployed on the kp.org Website in 2007. As of October 2009, 3.3 million members—38 percent of total members—had obtained user IDs and passwords to access secure features, including their electronic health records, on the kp.org Website. On average, almost 74,000 additional members registered to use the Website each month in 2009, and the great majority of those obtained password access to their health records. Accessing test results, securely e-messaging doctors, scheduling appointments, and ordering prescription refills were the most visited features during that time.

PHR Functionalities

KP HealthConnect's electronic member interface was fully deployed in 2007 and is linked directly to the EHR. Member online health services include the following:

- *Personal health record:* My Health Manager allows members to view most parts of their medical record, including lab results, immunizations, past office visits, prescriptions, allergies, and health conditions.
- *Electronic connectivity:* Members can send secure messages to their doctors, ask questions of pharmacists, and contact member services.
- *Online transactions:* Members can view, schedule, or cancel appointments, and they can refill prescriptions for themselves and other authorized family members.
- *Proxy access:* Authorized members can act on behalf of another family member (child or adult) to access online services.
- *Health and wellness:* Members may view health and drug encyclopedias, take a health risk assessment, get information about popular health topics, and use health calculators. Tailored behavior change programs for smoking cessation, weight management, nutrition, insomnia, pain, depression, and stress reduction enable members to actively engage in improving their health.
- *Health insurance management tools:* Members can use system tools to manage their health benefits, including estimating the cost of treatments and viewing medication formularies.

Clinical Decision Support

Kaiser Permanente developed evidence-based rules and documentation tools for physician and nursing workflows and embedded them in KP HealthConnect, giving clinicians easy access to evidence-based recommendations and decision support at the point of care. Expert clinicians from all specialties, regions, and health care disciplines are actively involved in the ongoing refinement of the clinical content.

Quality Improvement

Measurement and reporting of clinical data to improve quality and patient safety require identifying specific patient populations and documenting related clinical processes and outcome measures. KP HealthConnect provides data commonality that enables the organization to identify and share best practices across the organization, a challenge in the absence of a common platform. Kaiser Permanente regions generate a suite of standard clinical process and outcome measures on a regular basis at the clinical department or, in some cases, individual clinician level for management, improvement, or regulatory needs. In addition, Kaiser Permanente developed population management tools that extract data from KP HealthConnect to give primary care providers a comprehensive snapshot of their patients' preventive and chronic care status. This information, which can be sorted by the user in various ways, drives earlier outreach and intervention to improve preventive care and chronic care management.

CONNECTED FOR HEALTH

SECTION ONE

SETTING THE COURSE

CHAPTER ONE

OPPORTUNITY AND STRATEGIC LEADERSHIP

By Louise L. Liang, MD

Chapter Summary

This chapter describes the key leadership challenges involved in Kaiser Perman-ente's selection and implementation of a common electronic health record (EHR) system. It discusses the importance of a clear and compelling strategic goal, strong support and understanding from the board of directors, and full participation and buy-in from all leadership groups, especially physicians. It describes a unique "Blue Sky" visioning process that helped to establish broad principles for the transformation of health care quality and service—principles that would subsequently guide the implementation of KP HealthConnect. By bringing the entire organization together around the strategy, implementation planning, and execution, the KP HealthConnect initiative has helped forge a new, more collaborative culture throughout Kaiser Permanente.

Introduction

In 2002, pressure on the health care industry was increasing from multiple directions. Years of price increases that significantly exceeded the consumer price index were

Louise L. Liang, MD, is the retired senior vice president for Quality and Clinical Systems Support at Kaiser Permanente.

eating into company profits, robbing workers of salary raises and other benefits, and showing no signs of slowing. Compounding the frustration of employers, regulators, policy makers, and other stakeholders were reports that health care quality and safety were lagging behind other developed countries even though the United States spent significantly more on health care.

In 1999, the Institute of Medicine's report, *To Err Is Human,* concluded that tens of thousands of Americans were dying each year from preventable errors in the health care provided to them, and hundreds of thousands more were harmed or injured (Institute of Medicine, 2000).

In 2001, the landmark second IOM report on the U.S. health care system, *Crossing the Quality Chasm,* identified additional major problems in the American health care system, including delayed translation of knowledge into practice, ineffective application of technology, and inability to consistently deliver recommended care (Institute of Medicine, 2001). This second report touted information technology, notably the electronic health record (EHR), as a major solution for many of these failings. The report concluded that judicious use of information technology could help engage patients in their own care, prevent medical errors and duplication, offer reminders related to recommended care, provide the latest scientific evidence at the point of care delivery, streamline administrative processes, and enhance medical research.

Unfortunately, little improved with the release of these two IOM reports except for general awareness of care deficiencies. Frustrated with the health care industry, regulatory and accreditation bodies at the state and national levels moved to increase accountability by significantly increasing requirements for public reporting of clinical outcomes, patient safety metrics, and patient satisfaction.

At the same time, many large employers were addressing the increased cost of health insurance in their own way. Rather than paying the total cost for health insurance, employers were moving to insurance products that paid for only part of the cost by shifting a percentage of the premium to their employees, increasing co-pays for specific services, and adding deductibles.

All of these factors increased the out-of-pocket cost to the patient and put new demands on the Kaiser Permanente administrative systems to collect payment from each patient. These systems had always been considered low priority. Kaiser Permanente had pioneered comprehensive prepaid insurance, which required little or no additional claims for member payment, but our technology systems were not up to the task of administering these new complex insurance plans. With the significant revenue and customer service implications, it was important to collect these revenues promptly and accurately.

In addition, Kaiser Permanente had a long commitment and investment in improving clinical outcomes and patient safety through the development of evidence-based treatment guidelines. There was a shared belief between our health plan leaders and physician leaders that an EHR could make significant progress toward that goal by providing the latest science and clinical reminders at the point of care, enhancing knowledge, and decreasing human factors involved in medical errors.

However, despite excellent clinical outcomes, Kaiser Permanente was losing market share. There was hope that a comprehensive EHR would provide additional market differentiation on the basis of superior quality that would attract and keep members and provide the computer firepower to meet the growing employer demand for the administration of cost-sharing health plan options.

Given all of these pressures, in late 2002, George Halvorson, the new chairman and CEO of Kaiser Foundation Health Plan and Hospitals, set a goal to implement a more robust EHR than had been previously envisioned. What is more, he wanted to do it within three years, allowing some additional time for the two significantly larger California regions to complete deploying in the last of their many medical centers. Given that many single-hospital organizations took three years to complete a single EHR implementation, this was an unprecedented timeframe.

New Leadership, New Vision

Halvorson had arrived at Kaiser Permanente in May 2002 with a long history as an innovative CEO for Health Partners in Minneapolis, nationally known for its commitment to integrated quality care. His early leadership in the National Committee for Quality Assurance's development of HEDIS® (Healthcare Effectiveness Data and Information Set), one of the first tools to provide comparative measures of health care quality and service, was part of his legacy in improving health care at a national level.

One of the key reasons Halvorson accepted the position of CEO was his belief that Kaiser Permanente had the opportunity, and arguably the obligation, to leverage its integrated structure via an electronic health record. The physical and financial alignment of committed physicians, medical offices, hospitals, and prepayment to provide effective and efficient services would be facilitated by the flow of information through all parts of the organization.

Moreover, when Halvorson arrived at Kaiser Permanente, the organization already had an impressive history of innovation in health IT that reached back to the 1960s. This reflected the long-standing commitment of the physician leadership to using health IT to improve care. In fact, three Kaiser Permanente regions had received the coveted Davies Award from the Health Information and Management Systems Society (HIMSS) for implementing various forms of EHRs (Kaiser Permanente-Ohio in 1997, Kaiser Permanente-Northwest in 1998, and Kaiser Permanente-Colorado in 1999).

Over the succeeding years, Kaiser Permanente had evaluated various commercial EHRs and concluded that vendor products might not be able to support the size and complexity of the organization's more than eight million members, hundreds of medical offices, and eight regions. (See the "Kaiser Permanente at a Glance" sidebar.) Several disappointing attempts with small vendors in the mid-1990s confirmed these concerns. In addition, the only two American organizations of significant size that had deployed an EHR, the Department of Defense and the Veterans Administration, had internally developed systems.

Kaiser Permanente at a Glance

Kaiser Permanente, founded in 1945, is the largest not-for-profit integrated health care delivery system in the United States, serving 8.6 million members in eight regions (Hawaii, Southern California, Northern California, Northwest, Colorado, Ohio, Mid-Atlantic States, and Georgia). Members receive the entire scope of health care: preventive care; well-baby and prenatal care; immunizations; emergency care; hospital and medical services; and ancillary services, including pharmacy, laboratory, and radiology.

Kaiser Permanente comprises three entities: Kaiser Foundation Health Plans, Inc.; Kaiser Foundation Hospitals; and the eight regional Permanente Medical Groups. Together these three entities provide integrated care delivery through insurance plans; owned and operated hospitals and medical offices; and dedicated, prepaid, multispecialty medical groups. In addition, patient referrals may be made to non-Permanente community providers or non-Kaiser Permanente hospitals, as deemed necessary. Kaiser Permanente's mission is to provide affordable, quality health care services and to improve the health of its members and the communities it serves.

Facts and Figures (December 31, 2008)

- Total Operating Revenue: $40.3 billion
- Operating Income: $1.5 billion
- Capital Spending: $2.9 billion
- Hospitals/Medical Centers: 35
- Medical Office Buildings: 431
- Employees: 167,338
- Physicians: 14,641
- Nurses: 40,451
- Doctor Office Visits: 33.7 million
- Prescriptions Filled: 129 million
- Surgeries: 547,338

In 1997, Kaiser Permanente made a commitment to create an ambulatory, or outpatient, medical record system for all its regions. After several faulty starts, it settled on the approach of updating and expanding the Clinical Information System (CIS) developed internally by its Colorado region. Although delayed by one year and over budget, CIS had begun pilot implementation in Hawaii and was scheduled for deployment next in Southern California, Kaiser Permanente's second largest region.

Since the CIS project addressed only the outpatient medical office and had not kept pace with recent developments in the EHR vendor world, Halvorson asked clinical, operational, and IT leaders to re-examine the internal effort and compare it to "off the shelf" options that could provide additional functionality for administrative systems, hospital care, patient Internet portal options, and data capture and analysis. His objective was to have Kaiser Permanente reposition the initiative from a clinic office-based system into a program-wide strategic infrastructure that could leverage our integrated delivery system into a world-class national organization. The potential interruption of what appeared to be the final leg of a long EHR development journey created deep skepticism and angst. Further delays would be costly and frustrating, but Halvorson felt it was too critical to Kaiser Permanente's strategic agenda to proceed without thorough reassessment.

His experience with implementing and using electronic health records at Health Partners had convinced him that delivering quality care required a robust EHR. As he developed his agenda, he knew he needed to carefully reassess and reposition Kaiser Permanente's national EHR pathway and bring in a seasoned executive to be in charge of the project. He had been told by many inside and outside Kaiser Permanente it was important to look for an executive who could operate effectively in the complex organizational and consensus-driven culture that was the historical structure and operating approach of Kaiser Permanente, a national organization of eight semi-autonomous regions where strategic, budgetary, and care delivery discussions were often conducted on a regional, not program-wide, basis focused on local health plan and medical group issues.

Conveniently enough, the senior executive role with responsibility for the EHR effort, already established by Halvorson's predecessor, David Lawrence, included oversight for national performance in quality, service, and patient safety. Lawrence was trained as a physician and had been a member of the IOM task force that produced *Crossing the Quality Chasm*. He and Halvorson shared a deep understanding and commitment to leveraging health IT to improve health care.

When Halvorson called me to discuss a possible position on his new executive team, we focused on the oversight responsibility for quality and service, with only a brief mention of the EHR effort. I had operational experience in several similar integrated delivery systems, which included Harvard Community Health Plan in Boston and, most recently, Group Health Cooperative of Puget Sound in Seattle, where I had served as both COO of the insurance plan and delivery system and founding CEO of the affiliated medical group, Group Health Permanente. I was no stranger to significant organizational and cultural change. My experience included several financial turnarounds, driving cultural change to enhance performance, and serving as a member and chair of the board of the Institute for Healthcare Improvement (IHI), the internationally recognized leader in quality improvement headed by Don Berwick. He and I had started a long journey together in quality improvement in the 1980s when we practiced side by side as pediatricians and operating executives at Harvard Community Health Plan. As an added benefit, I was well known to Kaiser Permanente executives in both the health plan and the affiliated Permanente medical groups as a physician executive who was very familiar with the issues and challenges they faced. Although I had significant experience in the quality improvement area, it had always been as an operating executive. I had not held a staff position in over twenty years.

As the daughter of an engineer, my first love was math. Although I had learned computer programming for a summer job when I was sixteen, I had no professional experience in health IT. Unclear whether this was a good match with my experience, I called a long-time physician colleague, Jay Crosson, executive director of The Permanente Federation and a long-time advocate of the EHR efforts at Kaiser Permanente. The Permanente Federation supported the eight Permanente medical groups in national efforts, and he was very familiar with the issues. He assured me that overseeing CIS was not an IT job but an executive management job and reassured me that I should not be concerned. As it turned out, a few weeks before I arrived to join Halvorson's team in July 2002, he commissioned the EHR evaluation, jointly sponsored with Crosson, that would completely change the agenda of my work at Kaiser Permanente.

The Business Case and Board Involvement

In addition to putting together his senior executive team, Halvorson had helped make some changes in the Kaiser Foundation Health Plan and Hospitals Board of Directors, adding several seasoned health care executives, senior business executives, and consultants. They would be understandably rigorous in their review and oversight of the largest capital project in the history of the organization, an estimated $3.2 billion investment (a figure that grew to over $4 billion) over ten years for the initial implementation and ongoing maintenance of the EHR system. As Halvorson told the board of directors, it truly was a "bet the farm" decision for the organization and would provide major budgetary competition with the already significant investments needed for new facilities and seismically required enhancements for the California hospitals. Very few health care organizations had implemented electronic health records to the extent planned by Kaiser Permanente, and none had solid information on the value realized by their systems.

The business case was based partially on assumptions and experience from the Southern California region, and spotty reports of specific savings from outside organizations. In reality, the expanded, fully integrated EHR and related IT systems would support almost 80 percent of the clinical and administrative workflows in the organization, and no one could predict the full nature of the changes, much less the value, that could be gained. Making no assumptions related to increasing member satisfaction, competitive advantage, or growth, the conservative business case made a defensible case that the investment would break even and pay for itself in roughly eight-and-a-half years. Halvorson told the board that the actual payback would happen in half that time.

Make no mistake; this was a strategic decision, not one based on return on investment. The board of directors and the executive management of Kaiser Permanente believed that successful implementation and effective use of an EHR would streamline administrative and clinical operations and enhance performance in quality, service, and cost. The EHR would connect and leverage the Kaiser Permanente care delivery system via seamless information flow across all facilities. At the same time, it would connect to members via the Internet with features that could not be duplicated by its insurance or provider competitors. All of this was reflected in the project name, Kaiser Permanente HealthConnect.

The board gave KP HealthConnect much more than financial backing. It designated KP HealthConnect the number one priority in the organization's business plan for three consecutive years, and it linked the achievement of development and deployment milestones to every health plan and hospital executive's performance goals and compensation. Progress was reported to the board each quarter, and progress against plan was a condition for other capital expenditures, such as new facilities. This ensured that all of the key governance and executive leaders were fully engaged in this critical strategic endeavor. This large an endeavor in a three-year timeframe had never been attempted anywhere in the world, but the urgency was great and proved galvanizing for a new way of working to achieve this singular goal.

A Board Member's Perspective

When the board of directors blessed and funded the creation of KP HealthConnect, we saw it not only as a strategic investment in our competitive future but an affirmation of our brand. Kaiser Permanente was just developing a highly successful "Thrive" advertising campaign built around empowering individuals to manage their own health, and KP HealthConnect was a major means to that end. It was also the key to fully providing "patient-centered" health care and service, which would differentiate us in the marketplace.

This powerful combination of synchronized, real-time medical records to facilitate seamless teamwork between medical specialists and online access for patients to communicate with their doctor and view their own medical information has taken Kaiser Permanente health care into the twenty-first century.

In making this investment, the board saw it as a natural progression in fulfilling the promise of integrated medical care, a philosophy and a mission that

Kaiser Permanente pioneered and embodied since its inception. A company brand is a reflection of a company's mission and what it stands for, and KP HealthConnect has stayed true to that mission. When George Halvorson, the CEO, came to the board with the KP HealthConnect project, he warned that we were "betting the farm." In reflection, we were also betting that the Kaiser Permanente form of medicine is best for the health of our members and a beacon for the future of American health care. It turns out that was an excellent wager from the standpoint of a competitive market-place and improved medical care delivery.

The lesson here is a simple one: make decisions based on what is best for the patient, and you will be rewarded.

—Phil Marineau, retired CEO, Levi Strauss, and board member
of Kaiser Foundation Health Plan and Kaiser Foundation Hospitals, Inc.

All EHRs Are Not Created Equal

Even though there had been a long history of innovation and use of electronic systems to support care in various Kaiser Permanente regions, they varied significantly from each other and from KP HealthConnect in their functionality and capabilities. Some systems captured office visit notes by scanning and storing documents. Some clinicians entered data in their offices from notes made during the patient visit, and some accessed additional data drawn from other clinical systems, such as the laboratory and the pharmacy systems. None of the systems in use, including the CIS pilot, fully integrated all clinical information to provide a complete, real-time health record. The ultimate value achievable from an investment in health information technology is directly related to the breadth and degree of integration it provides across all parts of the health care delivery system. Only with significant levels of integration will health IT be able to address the gaps, errors, and duplication described in *Crossing the Quality Chasm*. Figure 1.1 schematically shows the health care system, the health IT functionality, and the benefits that can be derived. Although it is easier for large, highly integrated systems such as Kaiser Permanente and others, even individual practitioners can derive benefits from an EHR.

Selecting a Vendor/Partner

Although Kaiser Permanente ranks as the sixth largest hospital system in the country, none of our previous EHR efforts had included hospitals. Including them now was essential to the strategy to leverage the integrated health care delivery system via seamless information flow across all our facilities. In addition, increased understanding of hospital medication errors and other opportunities to deliver safer and recommended care made this a newly appreciated area of importance.

FIGURE 1.1. EHR FUNCTIONALITY AND BENEFITS.

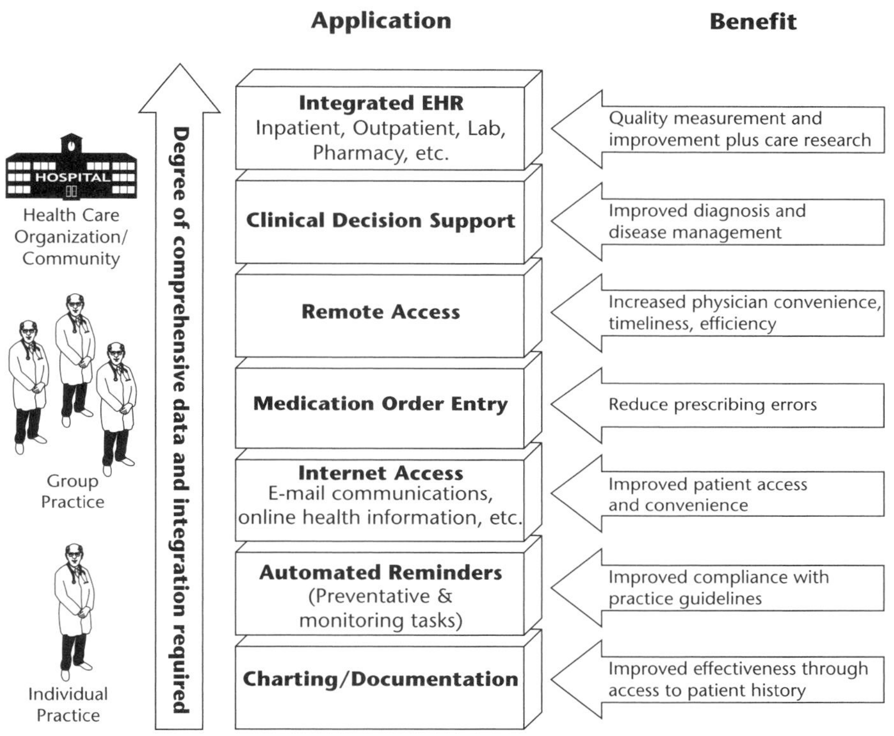

Application   **Benefit**

Degree of comprehensive data and integration required

Integrated EHR
Inpatient, Outpatient, Lab, Pharmacy, etc.

Quality measurement and improvement plus care research

Clinical Decision Support

Improved diagnosis and disease management

Remote Access

Increased physician convenience, timeliness, efficiency

Medication Order Entry

Reduce prescribing errors

Internet Access
E-mail communications, online health information, etc.

Improved patient access and convenience

Automated Reminders
(Preventative & monitoring tasks)

Improved compliance with practice guidelines

Charting/Documentation

Improved effectiveness through access to patient history

HOSPITAL

Health Care Organization/ Community

Group Practice

Individual Practice

Because Kaiser Permanente needed a system to support its hundreds of medical office buildings, dozens of hospitals, and online patient access for its more than 8.6 million members, there was a very short list of potential software vendors—essentially, two. One of them was the leading vendor for hospital systems but had limited experience with ambulatory applications. The other, Epic Systems, was the leading software vendor for ambulatory EHRs and administrative systems but had only limited experience with hospital applications. Neither vendor had fully implemented its integrated ambulatory/hospital/personal health record software in any health care organization. Neither had worked with a system as large as Kaiser Permanente, and there was uncertainty about whether the software from any vendor could be scaled to meet the demands of our size and multiregion structure.

Despite the fact that Kaiser Permanente's Oregon-based Northwest region was one of the earliest Epic clients, the competition was open and rigorous. The selection process was exhaustive, including site visits to health care organizations using the systems, such as Mayo Clinic and Geisinger Clinic, and multiple demonstrations with question-and-answer sessions between the vendors and our physicians, pharmacists, nurses, and IT experts. External benchmarking and the KLAS reports—the equivalent of the "Consumer Reports" for health IT—added comparative information. Hundreds of people were involved from throughout Kaiser Permanente over a period of six months. Everyone involved realized that this was unlike previous "bake offs," as these vendor selection processes were often called. Given the magnitude of the investment, the comprehensiveness of the software platform, the level of visibility, and high-level support, there would be no second chance.

Ultimately, Epic Systems was selected, despite its lack of hospital experience, on the basis of user satisfaction with its ambulatory medical record and administrative systems. In addition to a strong preference for Epic by the physicians and the medical group leadership, Epic's leadership demonstrated a deep understanding of health care delivery and a forthrightness even when their product did not deliver a requested function or feature. That characteristic would prove to be a helpful discipline when internal stakeholders wanted to customize the software, even when it was already proven to be highly functional for dozens of other organizations.

Start with the End in Mind

When an organization makes a strategic investment of the size of KP HealthConnect, it had better have a good understanding of its strategy at the beginning. The primary goal of KP HealthConnect was lofty: to transform care and service delivery. But what did that mean? I learned from my experience as an operating executive the importance of developing a shared vision. In this instance, what was the organization's vision of health care in the future? Even before the software contract was signed, the process to develop a shared organizational vision was begun.

As in all major Kaiser Permanente initiatives, the support and leadership of the Permanente medical groups was critical to success. I would work closely with a Permanente Federation physician executive who would engage and represent the eight independent regional Permanente medical groups. I knew and respected Andy Wiesenthal, the associate executive director for the Permanente Federation, who had extensive experience from leading the Colorado EHR development and CIS. Together, we would provide leadership for KP HealthConnect.

I relied on my intuition as a pediatrician, my experience as a health care executive, and my knowledge of quality improvement to develop the process. To me, quality improvement means data-driven and patient-focused decision making, respect for front-line knowledge, and profound knowledge of systems thinking. My job was to identify and frame the important questions and issues and then design and facilitate a process that engaged the right people with the right information to develop the right answers and solutions.

The Blue Sky Vision

In the first part of the process we brought in a group of people to develop the key themes. I wanted the wild and crazy thinkers in the organization—the ones that make us a bit uncomfortable, but we are smart enough to keep them around. They were the folks who were always pushing at the edges. We cross-cultivated those sixteen people with seven outsiders. The reason for the outsiders was to avoid group think, because I was concerned that Kaiser Permanente was a very internally focused organization. These guests represented expertise in technology, health care policy, economics, alternative delivery systems, and self-care.

The themes that emerged from what we called the "Blue Sky Vision" process—the name suggested open-ended vistas—were developed using a technique about which I was initially skeptical. Facilitated by both Robert Mittman, from the Institute for the Future, and graphic facilitator Tom Benthin, small teams wrote actual skits which they acted out for the rest of the group. It was very entertaining, but it was also eye-opening. Even though each team had totally different care delivery settings to visualize—the emergency room, chronic care, acute care, home, and so on—the themes that emerged were the same. They reflected the organization's aspirations, if not actual practices. They felt right and touched a nerve in a positive way.

I didn't know beforehand what those principles or themes were going to be. I was an observer at the back of the room. Strategic vision actually lives within an organization. Processes like this, if done well, will surface, articulate, and codify them.

The assignment was intentionally broad in nature. The object was to create a Kaiser Permanente model for health care delivery in 2015 to guide the deployment of the integrated EHR. There were only two constraints put on the group: the assumption that Kaiser Permanente would be a viable organization delivering health care in 2015, and that affordability of services was a consideration. The year 2015 was selected for a reason. Planning twelve years out took our technology readiness concerns and other common short-term barriers to major change out of the equation. Conversely, the timeframe was short enough to ground participants in developing achievable care delivery models.

As with health care experts across the nation, there was a diversity of views among the Blue Sky participants on the future of the health care industry and the specific implications for Kaiser Permanente. Some painted a dark picture of uncontrolled infections sparked by bio-terrorism and a collapse of health care financing due to severe economic depression. Others were more optimistic, seeing a continuation of the significant improvements in overall health care in the past fifty years. Participants were asked to identify the major trends affecting the health care industry. The group cited trends that are common to many discussions about health care's future. The list included continuing cost pressures on both employers and providers, changing demographics affecting consumer trends and workforce availability, a perceived infinite consumer demand for the latest technological services regardless of cost, and the continuing advances of medical knowledge that will turn many fatal diseases into chronic illnesses. The year was 2003, but it could have been today.

The process was framed to elicit multiple alternatives for care delivery, but what emerged from the group was a single, dominant model that placed the consumer or patient at the center. Prompting that consensus was a shared sense that many consumers—especially those with the means and choices—would demand a central role in managing their own care. An aging baby boomer population would put greater demands on the health care system than any generation before them, the group concluded, thanks to medical advances that would allow them to live longer while managing multiple chronic diseases. In addition, an increasingly diverse patient population with a wide variation in language, religion, culture, technology-based communication skills, ability to pay, and interest in alternatives to the traditional delivery model would require customized treatment.

This new paradigm would require the patient and the care giver to reassess their roles and responsibilities. For the patient, it would mean going beyond choosing insurance coverage to selecting individual sets of services, both in terms of medical care and wellness activities. For the clinicians and staff, the changes would require a fundamental shift in the way they view their relationship with the patient. Instead of the role of definitive expert, they would become coach and facilitator. The Blue Sky Vision concluded that in 2015 a successful health care organization would recognize that the *true* primary care provider has always been the patient and his or her network of family and friends. The patient's home would be the center of early diagnostics and service, with care givers serving as advisors on service options, clinical efficacy, genetic profile influence, and cost considerations.

The Blue Sky Vision, they further concluded, could be achieved with technology that already existed, including long-standing technology such as the telephone. The tricky task was to avoid falling too easily into the trap of uncritical adoption of technology and neglecting the hard work of leveraging that technology to achieve real change in care delivery.

FIGURE 1.2. THE BLUE SKY VISION.

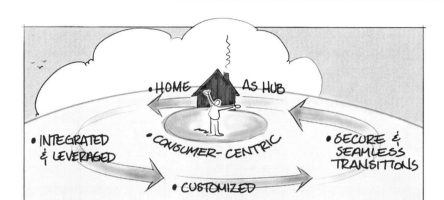

Four themes composed this new vision of health care delivery in the future:

- *Home as the Hub:* The home and other nontraditional settings would grow significantly as locales of choice for care delivery, and a patient's care delivery team would expand beyond the physician and other traditional care givers to include other community and family resources.
- *Integration and Leveraging:* Medical services to combat disease would be integrated with wellness activities to enhance overall quality of life as well as prevent and stem the onset of disease. Information technology would provide the vehicle to enable the leveraging of specialized clinical resources and increase patient and family involvement in care.
- *Secure and Seamless Transition:* Technology would allow the care giver to provide better informed and more efficient care to each patient. The computer would not replace human interaction, but enrich it by full availability of integrated longitudinal patient information coupled with the best knowledge and recommendations science could offer.
- *Customization:* Patients would become true partners in their health. Customer-centric care would be at the patients' convenience and customized to their specific health status and personal preferences, leading to a deeper understanding by patients of the care they are receiving and a stronger relationship with their clinicians.

Once the four themes were identified, another set of Blue Sky participants—these from the operational side of the organization—took up the assignment of identifying the range of practical and actionable steps and technologies that would change processes and mobilize the Kaiser Permanente workforce to achieve significant progress on the Blue Sky Vision within five years (by 2008). These phase two participants consisted of about ten of the original insiders from the first group for continuity, supplemented by a new group of our operational leaders. It was made very clear to this second group that their job was not to change or approve the themes that the first group had developed. Their job was to identify how to put the Blue Sky Vision into practice. They discussed operational implications for Kaiser Permanente across five categories: business and clinical processes, technology, information and knowledge management, facilities, and people.

Their operational imperative was to make this new era of care delivery as simple, seamless, and intuitive as possible for the patient. It recognized the patient as leader and/or partner in deciding his or her care and the home as the center for much of the care delivery. It also recognized that in the future, care givers would need to adapt to the patient's preferences for receiving information either electronically, by telephone, in person, or all three, depending on the nature of the information. And they would need to share, if not relinquish, the reins in deciding on the patient's health care path.

It also meant more than lip service to the age-old effort to move away from the departmentally siloed approach to medicine. In this new world, geographic as well as departmental and professional boundaries would be eliminated, and gathering and viewing data would not be enough. Interpreting and leveraging real-time and longitudinal information would be required to meet the specific needs of patients, whether they were in our facilities or at home, school, or work.

Once the Blue Sky Vision and its key tenets were codified, they were reviewed and discussed with the board of directors and the organization's key leadership groups, including Halvorson's national leadership team and the presidents and medical directors of each Kaiser Permanente region. The themes resonated, especially "Home as the Hub." The KP HealthConnect team would use these themes to guide the implementation.

In almost all other spheres of business and industry, electronic information systems coupled with the Internet have driven fundamental shifts in how business is conducted. Health care should be no different, but that has rarely been the experience with health IT.

We knew that KP HealthConnect could be the platform to achieve the Blue Sky Vision. With the immense changes required of clinicians and staff just to implement the EHR, could we also make fundamental changes in care delivery? It would be the only way to avoid adding cost and complexity to the system, but it is usually where organizations lose energy. That would be the key to achieving the Blue Sky Vision via KP HealthConnect, and we would need to stay focused.

Structure, Process, and Strategy

In his book *The Innovator's Dilemma*, Clayton Christensen talks about the challenge successful organizations have in innovating, or creating a product, or operating in a way that is different from the current successful products or culture. Christensen states that "[w]hen new challenges require different people or groups to interact differently than they habitually have done—addressing different challenges with different timing than historically had been required—managers need to pull the relevant people out of the existing organization and draw a new boundary around a new group. New team boundaries enable or facilitate new patterns of working together that ultimately can coalesce as new processes—new capabilities for transforming inputs into outputs" (Christensen, 1997, p. 175). Such teams were initially described by Steven C. Wheelwright and Kim B. Clark and dubbed "Tiger Teams" (Wheelwright and Clark, 1992). Only in hindsight did I realize that we had developed a Tiger Team perfectly designed to lead the changes needed to implement KP HealthConnect effectively.

When he joined the organization as chief information officer in 2001, Cliff Dodd established a set of principles to guide major national IT investments that would prove useful in the EHR assessment, the software selection process, and the structure of the KP HealthConnect implementation process. The five guiding principles were (1) common platforms, processes, and services should be adopted to achieve efficiencies; (2) it is better to buy an established product than to build a custom product; (3) integrated applications have an advantage over multiple applications from different vendors; (4) an application will suffice if it meets 80 percent of the needs; and (5) the customer/business must lead the work and be supported by IT.

These principles would serve Kaiser Permanente well to avoid pitfalls that had contributed to delays and frustrations in previous undertakings, where too much customization had blocked the ability to share applications between regions and where IT professionals had too often attempted to guess at the real needs of their clients without having deep experience or knowledge of their work. Avoiding these pitfalls was especially critical because most health care delivery processes tend to evolve over time with local conditions rather than being systemically designed, standardized, and documented.

During the EHR assessment and software selection, Dodd and I had shared oversight for the process on behalf of the health plan and hospitals. But as the new national team was formulated, it quickly became apparent that shared responsibility, or matrix management, would be a setup for confusion, misunderstanding, and delays. None of these would help in making the myriad decisions and aggressive timelines necessary to be successful. In keeping with his own IT principle of having the customer/business owner lead IT projects, Dodd agreed that I should have sole accountability to the CEO and the board of directors regarding KP HealthConnect.

With my experience as an operating executive, I could serve as the surrogate of the care delivery system and ensure that the operating and clinical leaders were engaged throughout the implementation. The core IT departments would provide technical staff as requested by my lead project executive, Bruce Turkstra. With a new team, new team leadership, clear boundaries, and permission to operate as needed to accomplish the implementation, we had our own Tiger Team. We were ready to go.

Implementation

Turkstra and I knew that the national KP HealthConnect team would have to operate in a more streamlined and efficient way than many were accustomed to in order to meet the aggressive timeline. His background as a partner at a major consulting firm had instilled unwavering commitment to understanding and meeting client needs. "We can't get that done" was simply not part of his vocabulary. The national team's role was to ensure every region's successful implementation. This included the development of capabilities in each region to sustain KP HealthConnect and its users long after completion of the software deployment. I frequently said that it was the national team's job to work ourselves out of a job. Regional success would be our only measure of success.

As we built our leadership team, Turkstra and I looked for leaders with a combination of knowledge of the health care delivery world and technical understanding and skills. The non-IT business owners included many nurses, physicians, and clinical technicians who brought their experiences caring for patients to the task. The team quickly developed processes that demonstrated our understanding of our regional customers and our commitment to make them successful. Our behavior spoke volumes in a way that the regions quickly recognized was a different way of interacting with Kaiser Permanente's national office. We made frequent regional site visits, held conference calls, shared decision making, and named dedicated regional liaisons charged with understanding regional needs and solving their problems.

The national team rapidly developed mottos that reflected our values and were used frequently to remind everyone of the priorities for the project. These included "Whatever it takes," "Our only success is regional success," and "Any regional problem is our problem." Every team member would have to deliver every time, on time, for the implementation to be successful. Some of the KP HealthConnect IT experts were veterans of previous efforts, but many were new to the project. Over time, the KP HealthConnect project recruited many of the best and the brightest within and outside the organization to our mission and our high-performance culture.

While the special status and organization of the KP HealthConnect team outside of the rest of the IT structure was critical to the success of the implementation in the given timeline, it caused friction and occasional resentment from the IT staff embedded in the old culture, with its lengthy processes for every decision or action. It would be important to help them understand how they could support this essential IT platform for long-term enhancement and maintenance without losing the positive aspects of the project's culture.

Early on, it became clear that the implementation would raise numerous procedural and policy issues. If the timeline was to be met and multiple regional solutions avoided, new ways of addressing these issues would have to be devised. Coordinating across regions and with other national initiatives was critical. One example was the establishment of the Joint Operating Group (JOG). In addition to the national KP HealthConnect team leader, Turkstra, and the project CFO, it comprised senior operational leaders from key national programs such as human resources, finance, IT, the Kaiser Permanente labor-management partnership, medical groups, products and marketing, and operations. JOG met weekly to address issues related to the project. When this group could not quickly clarify accountability and a pathway for resolution, our national executive sponsor group met to reach resolution. The executive sponsor group included me, Wiesenthal, the CIO, the CFO, and the national senior vice presidents of human resources, marketing and sales, and operations. Recommendations requiring our approval or clarification of accountability were dealt with typically within the week. Merely scheduling a meeting of these executives would have taken longer than a week in the usual processes of day-to-day business.

There was no precedent, no blueprint, for a venture like KP HealthConnect. In fact, it might have been exactly such uncertainty that set the stage for the old paradigm of eight siloed regions with a loose relationship to national functions to shift to a much more collaborative model. Now, the regional project teams looked to the KP HealthConnect national team to help them achieve a successful implementation by providing processes and expertise that accelerated problem solving and the sharing of knowledge from region to region. Whereas regional size (number of members) had been the historical currency for leadership in the organization, experience with KP HealthConnect became the new lever, and one of our smallest regions took the lead and taught everyone else on the basis of its experience as the first implementer.

A New Approach to Budgeting

The KP HealthConnect budget was also restructured to provide more national oversight and control than previous efforts. Traditionally, each region was responsible for all IT expenditures, including all regional and national IT priorities; ongoing IT maintenance; and mandates, such as regulatory changes. In addition, the regional IT budget competed with all other regional needs and agendas beyond IT for both operating and capital funding. With pressure to keep our insurance premiums down and to improve services and satisfaction, competition for resources was intense. The regional temptation would be to lengthen the KP HealthConnect implementation timeline or decrease funding for staff to develop the system, participate in national meetings, and begin system training. Skimping on workspace renovations, ergonomic mobile carts and computers, and IT enhancements and infrastructure could equally jeopardize success. Even with a well-designed system, poor user experiences during implementation could doom adoption or result in ineffective use of the system. Many health care organizations had foundered or failed because of these issues. Therefore, the KP HealthConnect project budget included all national and regional operating and capital expenses related to implementation.

Each year our national KP HealthConnect team and each of the regional project teams prepared budgets that were integrated and reviewed by the KP HealthConnect executive steering committee, composed of senior national and regional executives. Once approved as part of the organizational budget process, project leadership reviewed regional expenses charged to the budget to ensure their relevance to the project and occasionally offered advice, but otherwise all relevant expenses were booked to the national project budget. Saving money in the KP HealthConnect budget was encouraged, but missing deadlines and goals was unacceptable.

Acting in a New Way

A long-time colleague and friend of mine, Goran Henriks, talks about transforming health care to audiences all over the world. Henriks knows what he is talking about as the chief executive of learning and innovation for Jonkoping County, Sweden. Sweden has some of the best clinical outcomes among developed countries, and Jonkoping County is the best-performing county in Sweden and gets better every year. They achieve remarkable outcomes at a lower cost than the average Swedish county, obviously much lower than U.S. costs. Henriks' premise is that vision and slogans are fine but the experience of acting in a different way is what really changes people's thinking. He teaches that you help people change by providing an opportunity for them to act in a new way. The KP HealthConnect implementation gave us that opportunity, as nicely illustrated in a communiqué to me from one of our consultants, Richard Fitzpatrick, PhD, of Fitzpatrick Consulting:

> I think the tipping point may have come at a retreat I was helping to facilitate in Sonoma, Calif. It was still relatively early in the deployment process and the KP HealthConnect leadership team had gathered with a group of Kaiser Permanente physician leaders who had designated responsibilities for supporting the implementation process. It was a group of about 40 people grappling with the complexity and the fragility of how they would align the eight regions and their physicians around a shared approach to certain aspects of the deployment.

Then it happened. A physician stood up and said, "You know, up till now the rule was that everything varies unless you could make a compelling case that something ought to be standardized, and that was fine. Until now. From here on the rule is that everything is standardized, unless you can make the case that it ought to vary!" At that moment, the group collectively stepped into a new mental model. It was a new paradigm, and everything was changing.

One could argue this epiphany was the breaking through of a cumulative series of conversations over some period of time. KP HealthConnect leadership had become increasingly clear that unnecessary variation would add cost and cloud the Blue Sky Vision. Variation had simply been accepted as the norm and had been tolerated silently. It was a "simple rule" that was now being openly challenged. Doctors and managers had issues with a thousand things regarding KP HealthConnect, but the real underlying struggle was always about giving up something in order to get something. It was all about moving "from me to we" and sacrificing some individual clinical autonomy and customs, as well as some regional organizational autonomy, for the sake of the common good.

Lao Tzu's Chinese proverb rings true: "When the best leader's work is done the people say, 'We did it ourselves!'" Framing and facilitating a complex process involving significant change is leadership aikido. Never resist resistance. The journey begins with a compelling and personalized value proposition. Whether I'm a regional executive, or a physician toiling in the trenches, I want to hear a really good answer to the question, "What's in it for me and what's in it for us?" If that answer is compelling, I'll be more likely to engage in all the trouble and hassles it takes to get to that Promised Land.

So What's in a Name? A Microcosm

One of the project's first tasks appeared deceptively straightforward: name the system and develop communication materials to inform physicians and staff about its scope and implications. Supported by experts in branding and communication, the process initially went smoothly. That is, until the regions heard the expectation that the EHR name and communication materials would be adopted uniformly by all regions. Most of the regions had a long-standing name they used for their medical records tools. For example, Kaiser Permanente-Ohio's was called MARS, Kaiser Permanente-Mid-Atlantic States called its system PACE, and Kaiser Permanente-Northern California's system was named CIPS.

Why did it make any difference if the regions each used their own names, they asked. Some of the old regional names were used externally with patients and members, and wouldn't a name change cause confusion rather than clarity? How would they deal with that? The generic communications materials developed by the national project team used terms and references that were different from those the regions used. They wouldn't make sense to the regional physicians and staff, they argued. Why did they need to be the same? Was it really more efficient to develop them centrally?

In the past, several possible outcomes would have been likely. The national leaders could be dogmatic in the need to use the name and identical materials, in which case regional compliance would range from minimal to begrudgingly complete. The national team could back off, and the organization would encounter regional variants, complexity, and confusion for years to come. Or a compromise could be brokered, but each party might find the result unsatisfactory.

The challenge was to find a way to be adaptive and agile in meeting regional needs while furthering the overall purpose to develop a shared national IT infrastructure and operating platform. The issue of a single name for the system was a microcosm of much larger issues that we would face in the implementation. It would arise in software configuration, evidence-based clinical reminders and guidelines, the look of the computer screen, and response times to online member messages. The name was just the beginning.

A single name for the new system was non-negotiable. The formal naming was a step in reinforcing that this would be one system for all of Kaiser Permanente—a message that we were working to build something together—not for each region or department, but for all parties. But such operational issues had been left to regional discretion in the past, and in the two large California regions even delegated to their dozens of medical centers. Variation was the norm, not the exception. Mechanisms and processes for developing a single standard or making decisions about such standards across Kaiser Permanente were not even well established in most areas. It was often unclear which leaders or leadership groups had authority to make organization-wide decisions. There is an old Kaiser Permanente saying that carries the ring of truth: "No one is either so high in Kaiser Permanente they can make a decision, or so low they cannot veto a decision."

Seeking the balance between expediency to meet timelines and making change manageable without compromising the goals, the national team redefined its role and expectations with the regions. The national team would develop core templates for the regional teams to adapt as needed for local terminology and circumstances. This would result in clarity regarding shared uniform names and terms, as well as efficiency and relevancy in the development of region-specific materials.

The approach that the brand and communication staff used was respected for the rigor of the process, so when the name and logo were selected, most fell into line. The fact that we trademarked the name and logo was also a sign that we were serious. But it may be worth noting that even after agreeing to adopt the KP HealthConnect name, some regions added their own "taglines" for regional identification—a way of working around the name/logo and transitioning from names and terms that had been familiar in the region. Eventually many dropped these, probably discovering that the change was easier than anticipated.

The act of naming the system began to bring people together, even if unconsciously at first, around the reality that this was something we would share—something that would require us to act differently than we had in the past, because no one party would own it alone. Since then, KP HealthConnect has come to represent the shared clinical and business systems that support the daily office and hospital practice. The name, developed to reflect primarily the connection of clinical care among clinicians and with patients, also reflects the connection across the parts of our organization.

Connected at the Hip

KP HealthConnect encompassed multiple new software applications for each of the eight regions. This included as many as six major applications for the regions without their own hospitals and thirteen major applications for those with hospitals. Although there was initial complaining and chafing that each region would be interdependent with its fellows, the magnitude of the undertaking and the organization of the national team fostered new ways of acting to cope with these challenges. With the compressed timetable and multiple applications, there were bound to be conflicts in the combined schedules. To start, each regional executive team identified overall sequencing and timing according to their strategic priorities and operational constraints such as renovations, equipment, and resources. Since an application go-live, as the initial use of an application is called, involved hundreds of technical and program staff, the national team could support only one regional go-live at a time. The KP HealthConnect executive steering committee had been populated with a long list of key national and regional leaders with the expectation that the main task would be to referee scheduling conflicts between regions. But that was never necessary. In every instance over the course of the project, the regions together with the national team sorted out the conflicts and made adjustments so that every region's needs could be met with the limited resources of the national team. Frequent conference calls, in-person meetings, and shared problem solving had created a shared understanding, trust, and mission. Give and take became the norm. In the peak implementation years, the national team was onsite supporting an initial regional application go-live every weekend except Thanksgiving and Christmas.

In addition, the practice of lending regional staff evolved as a mechanism for shared learning. During a regional go-live, it was typical to have staff from a region that had already deployed be available to support and teach the new region. Staff from regions with future deployments also came to help and learn. What may have started as a desperate attempt to make the unknown less daunting became a critical technical and moral support during the go-lives. Many of the same staff who had sat together to learn and configure the software rolled up their sleeves and helped each other through the crucible of the go-live. Each region built on the experience of the previous ones so that all benefited. This was a long way from the days of eight autonomous regions.

Eye on the Prize—Value Realization

From the very beginning, we focused on achieving value from KP HealthConnect. This began with the development of the Blue Sky Vision to define a shared direction. An extensive review of the literature and canvassing of other health care organizations that had made similar investments revealed only anecdotal and fragmented evidence of benefits. In addition, no one had extensive experience with the full range of integrated applications and functions that we intended to implement. The one thing we heard repeatedly was that focus and discipline were essential. Our rapid timeline to start implementation—fifteen months between vendor contract signing and initial implementation—prohibited major workflow redesign before implementation. This was complicated further by varying workflows between regions, medical centers, departments, and even individual physicians. In fact, the decision making for the shared software configurations would drive a significant increase in workflow consistency just by decreasing regional variation. Beyond that, Carl Dvorak, COO at Epic Systems, felt that extensive work redesign of care delivery was not feasible before implementation. He cautioned that we couldn't know beforehand how the system would change workflow and what opportunities would present themselves. Dvorak's voice of experience proved accurate in so many ways. Our aggressive timeline forced us to manage some change before implementation, but much more would follow for years after, and is still evolving.

We began building infrastructure in 2003 to support the identification, evaluation, and spread of improvements and innovations related to KP HealthConnect. We knew that there would be significant impact from KP HealthConnect, but not necessarily what or where, so with operational leaders we developed a set of comprehensive metrics to identify operational impacts. We knew that spread of improvements and innovation would be faster with rigorous objective quantification, and so we developed a skilled evaluation unit to work closely with the operating units.

One of the most influential studies evaluated KP HealthConnect's impact on our Hawaii region of 225,000 members (Chen and others, 2009). It showed a 26 percent decrease in patient office visits from the year before implementation to the year after implementation, as a result of patients having additional means of accessing their care givers. Almost evenly spread over primary care physicians and medical and surgical specialists, the shift in utilization is dramatic and has far-reaching implications.

Paradoxically, total patient interactions with their own physicians increased by 8.3 percent with the use of secure Internet messaging and telephone visits as new care options. Physicians and their teams would have the opportunity to redeploy time previously engaged in now-unneeded office visits to sicker patients with multiple chronic conditions.

Learning from Others

We also knew that we would need innovative skills to leverage KP HealthConnect, so we began working with IDEO, one of the world's best-known design innovators, to improve our health care delivery processes. They had worked with SSM Health Care in St. Louis, which was the first health care organization to win the Malcolm Baldrige National Quality Award. IDEO taught us to see our processes from the viewpoint of front-line staff, who knew what helped them meet patient needs and what got in the way. IDEO also helped us to look at our processes from the patient's and the family's points of view. Their techniques helped us identify gaps and overlaps in our care processes that were invisible to us before.

We also developed a quality improvement strategic partnership with Berwick and IHI in 2004 to improve care and service leveraging KP HealthConnect. Although the institute had been internationally recognized as the most influential organization in health care improvement since its founding by Berwick in 1991, health IT's impact on the delivery of care was new terrain for both of us. We learned from their deep experience with many other excellent health care organizations throughout the world to apply proven practices and to test and develop many new ones. We focused on using known tools for improving medication safety, such as learning from "near misses," as the aviation industry does. We explored the complex interaction of human behavior and the use of computer-generated alerts and reminders. All of our hospitals committed to IHI's "Saving 100,000 Lives" campaign to reduce medical errors (Berwick and others, 2006). The experience of learning with 2,000-plus hospitals around the country opened new doors to us for benchmarking and learning.

Focus on Quality Improvement

Building an infrastructure for quality improvement began with the development of an organizational dashboard for clinical outcomes, member service, patient safety, and resource utilization. The availability of trended, comparable quality data with external benchmarks would support the board's oversight role, management's operational accountability, and local improvement. It would prove catalytic and accelerate the accomplishment of Kaiser Permanente's goal to provide care at the top-10-percentile performance level nationally. After a national benchmarking process with the best organizations and theorists in health care, we developed a program to build leadership and staff capacity for performance excellence. We tapped national and international experts to teach our leaders and develop our own experts. The tools and techniques we developed and taught equipped our front-line teams to improve the quality of their work every day. Combined with organization-wide commitment to three-year goals, this capacity helped us to improve performance every quarter. In the HEDIS report on health plan quality for the performance year ending December 31, 2008, Kaiser Permanente regions ranked number one among all health plans in the nation for eight separate metrics. These metrics reflect excellence in the management of chronic diseases such as diabetes, cardiovascular disease, and asthma, as well as preventive care such as the immunization of children and cancer screening in adults. Most notably, Kaiser Permanente ranked number one in the nation for breast cancer screening, and all eight regions ranked number one in their respective geographic regions.

The Power of Evidence

Evidence is powerful and comparative evidence is even more powerful. It has become a cliché, but no less true because of this, that quality improvement requires measurement. Where quality data is publicly reported, hospitals and physicians are motivated to improve—this stimulus is professionalism, stimulated by healthy competition.

Most health plans have pretty blunt tools with which to influence providers—pay-for-performance and discretionary reminder systems among them. Kaiser Permanente has the unique advantage of being both a payer and a provider system, and potentially more connected to the physicians, nurses, hospitals, and other staff providing care to its 8.6 million members. But those more than 150,000 staff and providers are all in different regions with their own leadership, culture, and marketplace pressures, so the influence of the collective on innovation around quality improvement was not as powerful as many had hoped and believed, at least not until KP HealthConnect arrived.

A by-product of this patient-centered information system is a population-based database, empowering Kaiser Permanente to have the most extensive, most complete, and most accurate quality of care information of any health care system in the United States.

Thanks to KP HealthConnect, physicians now not only know what they need to know about each patient, but can measure their own performance against their colleagues across the organization on clinical quality, safety, efficiency, equity, and service. Not only does each hospital know its own rate of preventable adverse events and complications, but now they each can see the comparable data from every other Kaiser Permanente hospital. Experience in other sectors about this kind of public reporting is that it leads to improvement—and that has begun to happen within Kaiser Permanente, as well. In part, this is a natural human tendency to respond to data that is less than perfect. But within the Kaiser Permanente family of hospitals and physicians, there is another, intensely powerful dynamic—a hospital or medical center that is doing very well on a specific set of measures becomes a beacon to the others, and people begin to reach out and "shamelessly steal" from one another, as the quality leaders are now beginning to call it.

Now the widespread availability of comparative and credible data allows everyone to learn from one another and create a push to get to the best—everywhere and all the time.

It also allows more effective governance in quality and safety. The Quality and Health Improvement Committee (QHIC) of the board of directors is responsible for oversight of the hospitals and the overall quality of care, in partnership with the Permanente Medical Groups. Comparative and credible data enormously strengthens this function of QHIC and energizes the national quality effort.

It took huge interdisciplinary and cross-regional teams for the "collaborative build" and implementation of KP HealthConnect. That culture set the stage for the use of KP HealthConnect data to benefit the millions of Kaiser Permanente patient members, and to enable the thousands of Kaiser Permanente medical employees to feel ownership of quality of care and their ability to implement evidence-based improvement strategies that work.

This is a model we need as a nation to carry our health care quality to the next level:

- Data collected in the course of care;
- Clinical, not claims, data;
- Comparative and transparent reporting;
- A culture of collaboration and collegial competition; and
- EHRs like KP HealthConnect that are just what the doctor ordered to make that goal a reality.

 —Christine K. Cassel, MD, MACP, president, American Board of Internal Medicine and chair,
Quality and Health Improvement Committee, Kaiser Foundation Health Plan
and Kaiser Foundation Hospitals, Inc. Board of Directors

In 2005, we began our 21st Century Care Innovation Project with IHI's support, involving nine of our primary care practice groups. Some of these primary care teams consisted of a handful of doctors with their nurses and administrative staff. Some involved entire facilities with as many as eighteen physician practices and all of their clinical and support services. This work was guided by the key themes of the Blue Sky Vision: consumer-centric care, home-as-the-hub of care, secure and seamless transitions, integrated and leveraged resources and expertise, and care and services customized to each patient. Every design team included a patient member to ensure that we never lost sight of who we were trying to serve. Many of the changes they tested, such as scheduled telephone "visits," have been adopted in the rest of our delivery system and have served as a starting point for additional changes and improvements.

With surprising rapidity, our patients have seized new ways of receiving information, support, and care in the wake of KP HealthConnect. More than 3.3 million of our 8.6 million members are active users of our Internet-based supports and services, including over 48 percent of our members over age 65. Patient primary care contacts are now conducted 41 percent of the time via secure e-mail messages or scheduled telephone visits, according to internal data.

When we started the Blue Sky process, we thought that we would identify very advanced technological devices and completely new ways to deliver care. What we discovered was that all the approaches and equipment we needed to transform care and service were already in use—at least somewhere. KP HealthConnect added the technical platform and operational opportunity to rethink many of our historical approaches. The changes developed and tested by our 21st Century Care Innovation pioneers have demonstrated the power of information. Information shared among all care team physicians and staff has enabled every support and clinical team member to help care for the patient. Information shared between patient and care team has liberated patients from the limits of the traditional care delivery system and engaged them in managing their health care and, more important, their health. During the Blue Sky Vision sessions we learned a quote from the science fiction writer William Gibson: "The future is already here. It's just not evenly distributed" (National Public Radio, 1999).

Lessons Learned

Many of the lessons we learned in developing KP HealthConnect will be detailed in the following chapters. Here are some of the most important lessons related to leadership, organization, and strategy:

- *Leadership Sponsorship:* High leadership commitment demonstrated through funding, priority setting, and executive attention and incentives is essential to accomplishing the technical, programmatic, and cultural changes necessary in a major EHR implementation.
- *Shared Vision of Care Delivery:* The Blue Sky Vision provided shared goals for the implementation and use of KP HealthConnect and unified leaders, teams, and users alike. It guided software decisions, prioritization, further IT investments, and innovation in how we deliver care.
- *Strategic Investment:* Positioning KP HealthConnect as a strategic investment to transform care and service ensured that it would be taken seriously by operating executives.

- *Tiger Team:* Creating protected space within the organization via senior executive leadership, structure, and budget for the KP HealthConnect national team to develop new ways of working with the regions and new problem-solving processes made it possible to deliver on the aggressive timetable.
- *Essential Partnerships and Engagement:* There were many parties essential to our undertaking. Our experienced software supplier, Epic Systems, shared our goal to improve health care. Our physicians, nurses, labor partners, and all other staff engaged fully in the work from the beginning. The changes we made were only possible because of their support and commitment.
- *Practice Changes Culture:* The implementation of KP HealthConnect gave Kaiser Permanente an opportunity to develop a new way of working together, which changed the historically semiautonomous regions into sharing, learning partners linked by technology but, more important, by trust and a shared mission.
- *Parallel Investments:* Building infrastructure for performance improvement and innovation created focus and capability for value realization. Developing rigorous tracking and evaluation processes enabled us to develop, identify, and adopt innovations and effective new practices from the very beginning.

SECTION TWO

LAYING THE TRACKS

CHAPTER TWO

IMPLEMENTATION THROUGH COLLABORATION

By Donna Deckard and Pamela Hudson

Chapter Summary

This chapter provides an overview of the key factors integral to the successful implementation of KP HealthConnect and to the change in organizational culture that accompanied and enabled it at Kaiser Permanente. It tells the story of the design and implementation of KP HealthConnect, beginning in 2003, and highlighting the key success factors. Finally, it concludes with a number of lessons learned, many of which will be relevant to any health care organization considering a large-scale information technology (IT) implementation.

Introduction

Successful implementation of a health care information technology system derives from more than just the right hardware and software. Technology is only an enabler; it is the people using the technology who change how work is accomplished or how care is delivered. A new IT system requires new ways of working that are more efficient, more

Donna Deckard is founding principal of Deckard Design and Consulting; Pamela Hudson is program director, EHR Implementation, University of California, San Francisco Medical Center. Catherine Hernandez, vice president of corporate communications at Kaiser Permanente, also contributed to this chapter.

uniform, and more integrated. This chapter tells the story of how, through the collaborative process of designing and implementing Kaiser Permanente HealthConnect, the organization underwent a cultural transformation from inefficient variation to standardization, from independence to interdependence, and from eight different regional health care IT systems to a single, uniform system across the entire enterprise.

While Kaiser Permanente's regional structure may be unique, the challenges the organization faced in creating greater uniformity are common to many mid-sized and large organizations, most of which experience some degree of variability across organizational units. For example, even in a single community hospital seeking to implement a health care IT system, there may be ten general surgeons on staff, each of whom has a different way of treating patients and documenting the care provided. For this hypothetical hospital, the relevant lesson from Kaiser Permanente is that layering technology on top of ten different processes for doing the same thing will not improve work processes. Without addressing these differences in work processes and organizational culture (the way people relate to one another), technology will simply "electrify" the existing chaos.

The culture change that took place at Kaiser Permanente as a result of implementing KP HealthConnect has had a lasting impact on Kaiser Permanente operations. Many program leaders believe that the "coming together" that took place during the KP HealthConnect implementation helped set the stage for the organization's high-ranking 2008 HEDIS scores in clinical quality from the National Committee for Quality Assurance. Similar cultural changes are necessary in any organization contemplating a major health care IT overhaul. Such a change is not simply about IT—it is about *everything in the organization.*

In 2003, when Kaiser Foundation Health Plan CEO George Halvorson issued a mandate to the organization to implement a single electronic health record (EHR) system across the organization's eight regions within three years, most thought this would be impossible. At that time, there had been teams of people within Kaiser Permanente, both at the national and regional levels, who had spent years developing and implementing various EHR systems at the regional and national levels. Some were built on commercially available software; others involved internal development of proprietary software. As a result, there was significant concern about abandoning legacy systems that had taken years to develop, but that stood in the way of organization-wide uniformity.

To meet the CEO's challenge, we developed a collaborative design and implementation strategy, resulting in a fundamental shift in the organizational culture.

Keys to Successful Organizational Change

Many factors contribute to the success of a project as large as the KP HealthConnect implementation. However, we believe that a handful of issues were of critical importance. They include executive sponsorship and leadership, giving "ownership" of the project to the end-users (rather than to the IT people), having the right team of people carrying out the project, and customizing only as necessary.

Executive Sponsorship

Because of the broad scope of the KP HealthConnect project, sponsorship was required at the highest levels of the organization, both nationally and regionally. At the national level, Louise Liang, MD, a senior health plan executive, was named to lead the KP HealthConnect project. She was accountable for the budget and timeline and reported directly to the CEO and the board of directors. In addition, the Permanente Federation named Andy M. Wiesenthal, MD, a senior physician executive with a background in quality improvement and IT implementations, to partner directly with Liang. The health plan's chief information officer, Clifford Dodd, was also named as a sponsor to ensure that the IT organization's resources, systems, and processes were in alignment and would provide the necessary support for the initiative.

Ken Hunter, chief operating officer for Kaiser Permanente's Mid-Atlantic States region and the lead KP HealthConnect sponsor there, provided the following valuable perspective on the role of the executive sponsors:

> While the role of executive sponsor may not typically show up on the project plan for an electronic medical record implementation, it was a key ingredient in the successful deployment of KP HealthConnect. A project this size and complexity takes many twists and turns over its life cycle, and the executive sponsor is the one who must work with the larger organization when those turns threaten the success of the project.

> As an executive sponsor, my first task was to recruit a sound project management leadership team. KP HealthConnect truly required a cross-functional team with individuals from many parts of the organization, not just IT. Once the team was recruited, I spent a good deal of time understanding and monitoring the project's scope, timeline, and progress. Problems, including inevitable budget challenges, came up regularly, requiring my immediate help if the project was to stay on track.

> Major parts of the sponsor role included breaking down organizational barriers and seeking more funding for certain aspects of the project. I also spent a good deal of energy on communicating the project's vision, progress, and impact on the region's care delivery and business processes. Since our implementation was part of an integrated national effort, I spent time coordinating with our national team on timelines and project scope. One area not to overlook is regular communications to the senior leadership team, who have their own objectives and agenda, and to the

regional president, who would sometimes receive feedback from parts of the organization about the project's "adverse impacts."

As executives, we are often asked to chair a committee or sponsor a work effort with the expectation that it will take an easy hour or month of our time. Serving effectively as the executive sponsor of an EHR implementation is definitely not one of those tasks. It will take all your leadership skills and organizational authority to successfully fulfill the role.

Engaging the Labor Partnership

To complete the leadership team, it was important to involve representatives of Kaiser Permanente's labor union partners. In 1997, Kaiser Permanente established the Labor Management Partnership (LMP), an innovative working relationship between management and a coalition of twenty-six local unions, representing some 90,000 Kaiser Permanente employees. The LMP served as the vehicle for the involvement of labor in the implementation of KP HealthConnect. Since the implementation was going to affect almost every role in the organization, it was clear that organized labor needed to be involved in each phase of design and implementation. Therefore, when the coalition of labor unions suggested that a full-time staff person be assigned to work on the national team as labor's representative, we welcomed the addition. Each region also included union representation on its project teams.

Claudine Salama, the national coordinator for the Coalition of Kaiser Permanente Unions, provided the following perspective on labor's role in the implementation:

Early in the planning for KP HealthConnect, management realized that the success of the system rested with the system users. Front-line involvement was required to develop effective workflows or routine patterns of work. Engagement by the organization's unionized workforce in the system design would be indispensable.

The Labor Management Partnership (LMP) was extremely important and became an integral part of the success of this project. As a result of the partnership involvement, more effective training materials were produced, and user acceptance of the new technology was high because the people who would be using it helped build the system. Most important, our national partnership agreement provided protection for employees who were displaced by the new technology. Workers were assured continued employment if they were willing to retrain; if not, they were offered a severance package. By addressing these thorny issues proactively, workforce planning could occur openly with collaboration between labor and management. As part of the agreement, labor agreed to promote the project at all levels and ask workers to take on new tasks. The role of labor in the success of KP HealthConnect continues to evolve and thrive.

Realization Teams

As a framework for the national and regional KP HealthConnect teams, Dodd, the CIO, introduced the executive leaders to the concept of "realization teams" (Figure 2.1). The model clearly outlined that KP HealthConnect was not solely an IT project, but was to be jointly managed as a partnership between operational and business leaders and IT. The structure called for an operations manager (also known as the business process manager) and an IT project manager, who were to act as partners and report to a realization team leader, who reported directly to the executive leaders and sponsors.

After an extensive external search, Bruce Turkstra, an executive from PricewaterhouseCoopers and Accenture, was selected as the realization team leader because of his deep experience in managing large-scale projects. Additional leaders (including the authors of this chapter and Robert Goldstein, IT project manager) were selected from among the organization's cadre of experts in care delivery, operations, and IT.

Once the national team was in place, the regions chose the leadership and members of their own project teams. Most regions ensured that senior leaders were named as sponsors, and many asked their best people to leave their current roles to take

FIGURE 2.1. THE REALIZATION TEAM WHEEL.

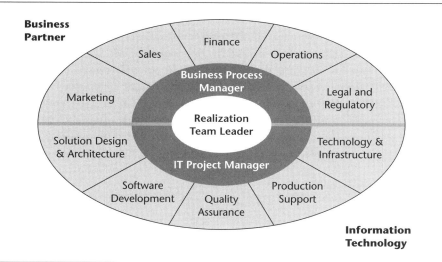

positions on the project teams. These staffing decisions, and leadership's commitment to them, were key factors for successful implementation in the regions.

Finally, it was critical that the EHR vendor, Epic Systems, be a full participant in the leadership team. Because of its vast size, the project was new territory for Epic. At the national level, Kaiser Permanente's executive team spoke regularly with Epic's chief operating officer, Carl Dvorak, and Epic's account managers were equal partners with Kaiser Permanente leaders. Epic representatives were included in all governance meetings, inter-regional meetings, and celebrations.

The Right Team

In his book *Good to Great*, Jim Collins writes that good-to-great leaders begin transformation by first getting the right people on the bus (and the wrong people off) and then figuring out where to drive it. The key to this is that the "who" questions come before "what" decisions—before vision, before strategy, before organizational structure, before tactics. Collins suggests three practical disciplines for being rigorous in personnel decisions: when in doubt, don't hire—keep looking; when you know you need to make a people change, act; and put your best people on your biggest opportunities, not your biggest problems (Collins, 2001, p. 63).

Because of the magnitude of the KP HealthConnect implementation, we did not have all the expertise we needed internally, and we anticipated that we would need many people during the peak implementation period who would not be needed later. We therefore contracted with a major consulting firm that had prior knowledge of our IT infrastructure and plans for time-limited expertise, and with another firm to provide qualified interim staff for backfill support during training and regional go-lives.

As the project moved through multiple phases each year, each phase required a re-examination of the people in the different roles. Many midcourse staffing changes had to be made along the way. In short, the people chosen to work on this type of effort have to be the best and brightest, and have to be flexible, creative, and able to work as members of a high-performing team. The project required working long hours, evenings, and weekends. In addition, to lead and participate in this effort, one had to have the tenacity to work in uncharted territory, have the confidence to find and lead the way, and be willing to take risks and learn as work progressed.

Balancing Enterprise Uniformity and Local Customization

In addition to strong leadership and staffing, another key to the successful implementation was flexibility. Although the goal was to move all eight Kaiser Permanente regions to a single IT system, the project leaders understood that forcing too much uniformity across the program would run into conflicts with unavoidable regional variation. Thus the design process created a "template" or standard core system that all regions would use as a starting point. Regions were permitted to customize that standard, but only if they would abide by two critical rules: first, the integrity of data had to be maintained at all times, and second, interoperability across regions had to be protected. These rules provided clear direction for all team members and helped clarify when customization was useful and when it would be harmful to the overall project goals.

The Collaborative Build

The size and speed of the Kaiser Permanente implementation was unprecedented. The project leadership team started with the philosophy that "no one size fits all," and that each region had unique needs. However, to achieve the long-term vision for the organization, success would be dependent upon more standardization. If each region designed and built its own system, it would slow down the process and increase overall cost. Kaiser Permanente had to approach this implementation as an entire system, not as eight separate regional systems. From this "systems" perspective, the concept of what we called the "collaborative build" was born.

The collaborative build was the process by which KP HealthConnect would be designed at the national level, with collaborative input from all the regions. The end result would be a system that could serve as a baseline for each region's implementation. The design issues (or software decisions) to be addressed as part of the collaborative build included, among others, configuration settings, clinical content, medical terminology, basic security, decision support tools, charting templates and tools, and standard reports. Several of these topics are explored in more detail later in this chapter.

First Standardize, Then Diverge

The idea for a Collaborative Build was itself a collaborative creation born of necessity (and about forty pads of that poster-size paper you can stick up on the walls). Epic's most experienced implementation staff worked with our new Kaiser Permanente and Deloitte partners to develop the approach and turn it into practice. KP HealthConnect presented a unique challenge in size, speed, and scope. It was possibly the world's largest and fastest EHR deployment, and they were also implementing Epic's integrated business applications for scheduling, registration, billing, and more—all at the same time. It involved four key objectives:

- Reduce the cost of unnecessary variation across regions;
- Create a platform to share best practices across regions;
- Preserve regional autonomy and innovation; and
- Meet timeline and budget goals.

The idea of the collaborative build itself was fairly simple: define what elements should be held constant across all regions to further the sharing of best practice and reduce unnecessary variation. List everything all regions could agree on and build that out first. Also, clearly define what would be managed regionally to meet local needs and avoid stifling creativity.

Ensuring that everyone involved understood one key concept turned out to be critical to our success: *diverging later would be easy, but converging later would be almost impossible.* Together, we continuously reinforced that point and helped people recognize the importance of initial standardization. Regions could always decide to do something differently later if it turned out to be critically important.

Once we got started, the teams noticed that the more they standardized, the more they could leverage work done by other regions. Over time, you could see people's minds shift to first think how they could standardize instead of why they might not want to. The collaborative build worked well and became standard operating procedure at Epic for other large multiregion health systems that followed, and at Kaiser Permanente for other large projects they undertook.

—Carl Dvorak, chief operating officer, Epic Systems

Goals and Assumptions

As noted in Chapter One, the KP HealthConnect design had to help the organization reach the future care delivery model described in the Blue Sky Vision. The design also had to support achievement of four established organizational goals, known collectively as the KP Promise: quality care, personalized care, convenient service, and affordability, as illustrated in Figure 2.2.

With these goals in mind, the leadership team made a number of decisions in advance of the design process concerning issues such as scope, scalability, and the number of software "instances" (or copies) of the program. These decisions and other baseline assumptions were considered in the system design, and they included the following:

- The project would include the full suite of Epic products, such as clinical systems for the medical offices and hospitals; inpatient and outpatient scheduling, registration, billing, and hospital pharmacy; Internet access for members and patients; and data warehousing and reporting.
- As shown in Figure 2.3, these new systems would be integrated with legacy clinical ancillary systems such as lab, pharmacy, imaging, and so on; insurance systems (benefits, claims, pricing, and so on); and financial systems (capital planning, financial reporting, and so on).
- All eight regions would implement the integrated system.

- Existing EHR systems would be replaced by the new system.
- A total of eighteen copies of software would be needed to ensure rapid response times for system users. The two California regions would each have six copies of the software, due to their large size.
- Differences in the physical layouts of hospitals and clinics would mean there would be few identical work processes across regions.
- We would have to deal with the fact that some regions owned and operated hospitals, while others contracted for these services.
- Patient access to the system would be through a Web portal that had already been developed on kp.org (see Chapter Eight).

FIGURE 2.2. THE COLLABORATIVE BUILD.

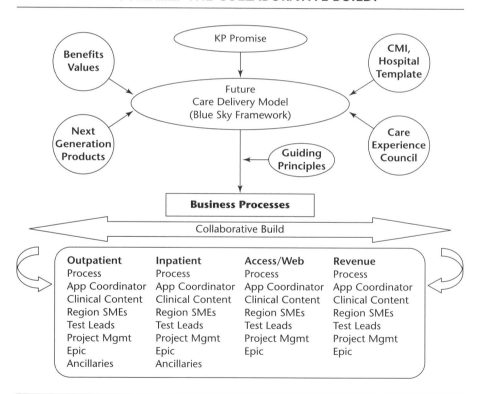

FIGURE 2.3. KP HEALTHCONNECT SCOPE: THE FULL SUITE OF EPIC PRODUCTS.

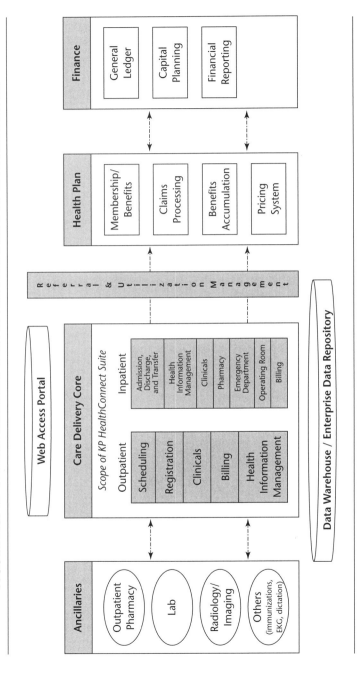

This list of "givens" seemed daunting, with many challenges inherent in each of the elements. This was more than just an EHR; it was a program-wide system that would integrate the clinical record with appointment scheduling, patient registration, and billing, and this information would be available to patients via the Internet. In short, this project would fundamentally change how almost *everything* was done in the organization. In fact, we estimated that 80 percent of the daily work at Kaiser Permanente would be affected in some way.

Design-Build-Validate Sessions

As the framework for the collaborative build, we used Epic's process of design, build, and validate (DBV) to develop the baseline KP HealthConnect system, including the evidence-based clinical content and tools that physicians and other clinicians would use at the point of care. This is a major undertaking for even smaller organizations, but in our case it had to be adapted to account for eight regions and all the different Epic products being implemented over a roughly five-year period (2003–2008).

"Design" refers to the decisions related to how the software would work, such as how data is defined; what data is collected and where it is recorded; how data flows from one part of the system to another; and what templates and special tools would be available to facilitate entering information, specific workflows for each software application, and integrated, end-to-end workflows across multiple applications. "Build" refers to the process of configuring the software to reflect these decisions. And "validate" is the process that checks to see that the software is performing as designed.

Ultimately, over 350 staff from all eight regions, specialty areas, and the national organization participated in nine two- to three-day-long DBV sessions over a period of three months. These groups made thousands of decisions, capitalizing on the wealth of technical and process expertise across the organization. This process had the following characteristics:

- Openness and inclusivity: operational leaders, content experts, clinicians, IT experts, and labor partners;
- Representation from the full spectrum of the organization: marketing, finance, patient safety, compliance, quality, operations, care delivery, and legal;
- Ability to gain support from leadership when needed to resolve stalemates, finalize decisions, and remove barriers; and
- Skillful facilitation to enable large-group decision making.

Start with the Foundation

The collaborative build included detailed design of a number of different functions and tools within the system. To give a flavor of the build, the following provides a deeper look at the design decisions made in few key functional areas: data standardization, medical terminology, and clinical content.

Data Standardization. Standardized data formats were critical for the organization to achieve its vision of enhanced care delivery through continual learning and improvement. Even seemingly simple data required review and new decisions. For example, there were more than 2,000 different types of office appointments across the eight regions. Many were very similar but not identical. Future analyses relative to patient access, comparative efficiency, and work load, for example, would be extremely complex if not impossible without significant standardization. During a collaborative design session involving operational leaders, IT, and content experts, we agreed upon approximately 250 appointment types that would be configured in the new scheduling system as the only allowable choices. Appointment types included the length of the visit and the medical purpose for the visit, and in aggregate they covered the dozens of different departments and medical and surgical specialists. Any changes would have to be reviewed and approved in a central process to manage the standardization and minimize the risk that variation would increase over time. In addition to providing a basis for evaluating performance and identifying best practices, the standardized collaborative build elements enabled data to flow between one part of the system and another and within the various regional copies of the national collaborative build.

Medical Terminology. One of the most challenging aspects of the collaborative build was embedding a common medical terminology into the new system. Prior to the collaborative build, Kaiser Permanente used a medical lexicon that was closely aligned with the Systematized Nomenclature of Medicine-Clinical Terms, or "SNOMED-CT"—a set of standard terms for medical data, developed by the College of American Pathologists. Although Kaiser Permanente's lexicon contained hundreds of thousands of health care concepts and had been developed over several years, this was the first time it was being used widely in active daily patient care delivery. During the collaborative build, thousands of additional terms were added to support operational needs, such as entering orders into the medical record and sending them to the appropriate department such as pharmacy, reporting laboratory and other test or procedure results, billing, and other recording of clinical events and care.

In 2003, the U.S. Department of Health and Human Services Office of Health Information Technology announced that SNOMED-CT had been licensed as a standardized medical vocabulary available for free use in the United States. As of 2007, the distribution of SNOMED-CT was made available worldwide. Kaiser Permanente continues to submit new terminology to enrich SNOMED-CT so other organizations can benefit from our efforts.

Clinical Content. The lifeblood of a health care IT system is the clinical content it puts at the fingertips of doctors and other clinicians. The software decisions and tools to support efficient and comprehensive recording of clinical information and the consistent use of evidence-based recommendations for prevention and the management of acute diseases and chronic conditions are called "clinical content." How these decisions would be made was critical to achieving the long-term vision of KP HealthConnect as the platform to enhance care delivery.

To develop clinical content for literally hundreds of topics, the collaborative build team established "communities of practice" for nurses, pharmacists, ancillary services, and physicians by specialty and/or care setting. Each group met intensively to make the initial software decisions and then less frequently, as needs evolved.

Communities of practice were given the following set of objectives:

- Use common data definitions and consistent data collection methods;
- Define where regional variation was acceptable;
- Establish best practice benchmarks;
- Define common performance measures;
- Incorporate quality and patient safety into clinical documentation and orders with alerts and reminders;
- Incorporate evidence-based medicine at the point of care to improve outcomes and reduce risk; and
- Facilitate the sharing of lessons learned and best practices to rapidly incorporate innovation across the program.

It was clear that the communities of practice could not be created by management edict. It was necessary to provide the right conditions and support for each community to grow and prosper on its own. Leaders carefully "sowed" each community with individuals who were passionate about technology and/or clinical care, set broad objectives, and allowed them to define their own work. Communities were nourished with summaries of research on best practices in their specialty areas, developed by the Kaiser Permanente Care Management Institute (CMI).

Each community of practice agreed upon the level of standardization judged necessary and feasible for their area. These collaborative decisions would be reflected in the software in various ways, including various Epic SmartTools (see Exhibit 2.1). As CMI staff described this work, "This means thinking about guideline content in a new way. Even though previous tools like pocket cards have aimed at making guideline implementation easy for clinicians, the process of creating SmartTools requires content experts to think in great detail about moment-by-moment flow of care within a clinic visit. At exactly what point in the visit should a statin (cardiac medication) alert appear? When the provider is reviewing the list of current medications? When he or she is signing off on any orders or plans? . . . With a solid understanding of the process of care, KP HealthConnect builders can begin to create documentation and decision support tools that support the process and reflect the evidence" (Woods, Licht, and Caplan, 2004, p. 58). In addition, an internal Web-based clinical library was created to improve the adoption and use of clinical content across regions. Using a search engine, a clinician could search content by type, diagnosis, author, specialty, or region and view the information online.

EXHIBIT 2.1. "SMARTTOOLS" FOR SMART CHARTING.

KP HealthConnect includes a variety of so-called "SmartTools" to help streamline clinical documentation and communication tasks. With SmartTools, clinicians can easily document patient encounters; code diagnoses and procedures; enter clinical notes; document telephone encounters; maintain problem lists; order laboratory and radiology tests; send prescriptions; and use the system to send and receive patient-specific messages, phone calls, and referrals. SmartTools include the following.

SmartSet   Allows clinicians to document all aspects of a patient encounter on a single form from which they can place orders, assign diagnoses and levels of service, complete progress notes, and much more.

SmartPhrase   Allows users to type a few characters that then automatically expand into a much longer phrase or block of text.

SmartLink   Retrieves and displays data maintained in the patient record.

SmartList   Allows users to enter information into a SmartText from a list of pre-configured choices. These are color coded and provide the following choices:
- Yellow = single
- Blue = multiple

SmartText   Consists of standard templates or blocks of text for use with a specific reason for visit, call, or contact. A template can contain
- Words
- Links
- Lists

OrderSet   Compiles groups of individual orders that are specially configured for a particular purpose.

Navigator   Provides a sequence of activities to assist with the process of
- Admitting
- Rounding
- Consulting
- Transferring
- Discharging

Some groups also focused on collaboration between nurses, pharmacists, and physicians regarding standardized data, clinical documentation, treatment protocols, and other clinical areas of interest. Many of these communities of practice have continued to provide direction for their areas and medical specialties.

From Design to Implementation

The collaborative build held its last session in September 2003 and completed testing in October 2003. The shift from design to implementation was a major milestone. The cultural change that took the organization from region-specific IT development to the collaborative build had a major impact on the way implementation was carried out. Instead of designing and building the system eight times, we could carry out parallel implementations in all eight regions. This was a major paradigm shift, as the model previously used for IT systems was for each region to independently design and implement in the first site, evaluate, make adjustments, and then move on to the next site. Had the organization stayed with this deployment model, KP HealthConnect implementation would have taken significantly longer. In addition to the national collaborative build, we adopted a standard implementation methodology aided by Epic's experience and advice. Multiple parallel implementations across the entire organization allowed us to learn across regions and begin achieving the benefits of a common system in a shorter period of time.

As noted earlier, the national collaborative build used a process called Design-Build-Validate. When it came time for the regions to take over and move into implementation, the order switched to "Validate-Design-Build" (VDB). The change in the order was not trivial. Regions would first *validate* the collaborative build to understand how the national model, which was uniform across all regions, would work for their region. They would then *design* and *build* only those additions or exceptions that were necessary given their business, clinical, and operational needs (for instance, hospital versus non-hospital-based regions, or the presence or absence of specific clinical departments). This allowed each region to use the national collaborative build and match their work processes and preferences to it, although designated parts of the software (master files, data fields, and processes) could not be altered.

With this standard approach in place, each of the regions began to develop its implementation strategy. The Hawaii region volunteered to go first. Prior to the KP HealthConnect project, this region had been implementing an internally developed product, known as the Clinical Information System (CIS). They had already deployed the system in almost 80 percent of their medical offices on Oahu and approximately 30 percent of the sites in Maui, as well as several specialty departments. When CEO George Halvorson made the decision to implement a single integrated system—KP

HealthConnect—in all regions, Hawaii made a bold choice to move to the new plat-form as quickly as possible.

The Hawaii region began deployment with their "go-live," as the initial use of a new application is called, in April 2004. Several more regional go-lives took place that year, and in 2005 and 2006 implementation was in full swing across the program. Once the California regions started to implement in their numerous medical centers, there was a go-live or software upgrade almost every weekend for two years.

Gladys Ching and Peggy Latare, MD, who helped lead the KP HealthConnect implementation in Hawaii, recalled the go-live experience for the authors:

> Looking back, implementing the KP HealthConnect at Kaiser Permanente-Hawaii was a turning point. We had partially implemented two EHR products before switching to KP HealthConnect, and many lessons were learned from that process. Technically, there were challenges to convert data from one platform to another, but those challenges paled in comparison to challenges faced by the clinicians in their daily work. These included overcoming fears of looking awkward or clumsy in the exam room with patients when trying to use the computer, while still ensuring positive patient interactions and high productivity levels. The ultimate challenge was learning how to organize and filter the clinical information to make a positive difference in the patient's care.

> It was an excellent lesson that change—even if it is considered positive—brings with it an adjustment period that includes a negative response in almost everyone. That negative response is followed by a realistic adjustment phase and, finally, acceptance and integration. This journey made it possible for us to transform the way we deliver care, including the use of non-traditional access (for example, telephone appointments and e-visits), making the integration of care that Kaiser Permanente is known for a technological reality.

Regions as Customers

In preparation for the regional implementations, the national team engaged the regions by meeting with each region's senior leadership team, conducting product demonstrations and assisting them in implementation team selections. In these early discussions, the national team exerted its influence, especially about project leadership, knowing that this was delicate territory. Since the national team was accountable to the CEO and the executive steering committee, it took its oversight role seriously and was very candid in its observations and guidance. These meetings set the stage for a new way of working between the national organization and the regions, and some of the core values that emerged were adopted by other national projects and departments.

Each regional visit was unique, and each region was in a different place in terms of its capability and readiness. Each region had wanted to implement the Epic products in a different sequence, on the basis of differences in their care delivery structures, operational strategies, and market needs.

As the project progressed, the volume of parallel regional deployments grew, and the number of people involved across the organization reached into the thousands. To establish a formal and ongoing engagement mechanism with the regions, the national leadership team created the position of implementation manager for each region. These implementation managers became the single point of contact for the region, responsible for ensuring that communication was sustained between the national team, the regional implementation team, and regional leadership. Together with Epic's implementation coordinator, the implementation managers worked directly with the regional leadership and team to monitor progress, identify and escalate issues, and ensure that necessary vendor and national resources were available.

Belva Denmark Tibbs, Kaiser Permanente-Ohio's vice president for medical operations, and Walid Sidani, MD, associate medical director for the Ohio Permanente Medical Group, compared the role to that of a house remodeling contractor in the following communication to the authors:

> Imagine you are renovating the kitchen and bathrooms in your home. Anticipation of the new state-of-the-art plumbing in the bathroom and technologically advanced appliances in your gourmet kitchen has you salivating. However, in order to finish the work, the renovation must occur during the holiday season when your home abounds with family and friends. That was the best metaphor we could use to describe the implementation of the KP HealthConnect ambulatory clinical system in the Ohio region. We often referred to the implementation manager as the contractor who was responsible for collaborating with us as we designed our future living space, identifying appropriate resources and best practices from other regions, helping us avoid potential pitfalls and, ultimately, overseeing the implementation of our plan.
>
> Like a skilled contractor, the implementation manager ensured that we were still able to provide quality care and service to our patients during the implementation process while living within resource constraints.

Communicating the Vision

For an organization with disparate regional structures that valued local autonomy, developing the collaborative build required a significant cultural shift. National and regional project leaders needed to clearly and consistently communicate the KP HealthConnect vision and its benefits for the organization, for members and patients, and for employees and physicians. Further, with the limited success of previous attempts at a common EHR system, project teams and the organization as a whole needed to understand how *this* project was different and *why* it was better positioned for success than previous EHR initiatives.

Several communication strategies were used to support acceptance and implementation of KP HealthConnect. A dedicated national communications team created a comprehensive communications plan including foundational positioning and core messages for the system. The plan included creating awareness, building knowledge, managing expectations, supporting superusers, enabling and motivating all users, and building proficiency. With help from Kaiser Permanente's public relations staff, the KP HealthConnect name was selected and trademarked, and a consistent look and feel was developed for printed materials that were shared with a network of regional communicators across the program. This approach connected all of the work visually and ensured that all regions were speaking consistently about their work and the end goal.

A centralized intranet site was also created to support project teams across the organization. The site prominently featured the KP HealthConnect goals and included product demonstrations and configuration documents, meeting schedules, regional project plans, and training materials accessible to all regions. The site also included a directory of project teams to facilitate peer contact across regions. As the project gained momentum, the site included regular leadership messages and project progress against milestones. The site was updated on a daily basis, and project teams received weekly e-mail newsletters with direct links to new Website content.

To further improve communication, coordination, and learning, quarterly inter-regional meetings of the national and regional project implementation teams and leadership were established. These in-person meetings helped to keep regional teams aligned around goals; build a community of knowledge; and foster inter-regional relationships, problem solving, and accountability.

In addition to the quarterly meetings, all project leads from the regions, the various support departments, IT teams, and the national team met once a year to determine the go-live schedule for the year. During this time, a master schedule was negotiated and developed. This regional interdependence created a sense of trust and accountability for everyone across the organization. Everyone realized that they played a part in sustaining the schedule, and if they didn't meet their deliverables it affected everyone. Not everything was perfect, and there were some schedule changes, but for the most part deadlines were met—an amazing feat for a project of this magnitude.

In the weeks and months leading up to each go-live, all regions executed various communication activities to prepare users for training and other launch-related activities. These included "talk shows" or videotaped sessions featuring operational leaders and project experts that were Web-broadcast during lunch hours; department meetings for front-line supervisors featuring product demos; and "forest and trees" meetings focused on both the high-level vision (the forest) and practical, hands-on demos (the trees). Other communication modes included newsletters, videos, Websites, and CD-ROMs.

User Training

The ultimate users of any EHR are the clinicians and staff. Readying them for system adoption is complex and requires significant training. In the beginning, much of the training material delivered to users was *system-centric*. It was designed and delivered by personnel who were experts on the KP HealthConnect system, not in operations or clinical care. The training materials described the system features and functions and told users how to access them. It soon became clear, however, that training needed to be *user-centric*. In other words, the training materials needed to focus on the users' needs and the specific tasks they needed to complete and then show them how the system could help them work more efficiently. This approach helped clinicians and staff learn and adopt the system faster. Users were given onsite training, time to practice with the new system both during and after go-live, and staff to fill in during training, all of which helped to ease the transition.

Clinician Adoption

No matter how effective the training, the natural reaction to change is resistance. Every individual has a threshold for how much change he or she can absorb. Implementing a complex EHR is not only technically difficult and operationally demanding, it involves introducing a whole new way of conducting and documenting the daily work of delivering patient care.

Many clinicians found these changes challenging. However, over a period of a few weeks or months, virtually everyone was able to order tests, write prescriptions, enter diagnoses, and manage patient e-messages. Naturally, full competency with the more sophisticated clinical content tools would be an ongoing task.

To accomplish this, clinicians were provided with a number of "self-service" training opportunities, ranging from Web-based tools and online help to the Kaiser Permanente *Blue Book for Charting Techniques*, a customized version of a generic book describing Epic SmartTools for clinical content. In addition to helping clinicians adapt their charting/documentation tasks to take advantage of the tools within the system, the *Blue Book* also helped them restructure their thinking to recognize the repeated use of a manageable number of charting concepts. As a result, they began to see the value in using SmartTools to quickly and comprehensively write a medical note with a few key strokes.

Over time, clinicians have used the charting tools mostly as they were designed. Some have been modified to reflect personal preferences, and new tools have been created from scratch. Best of all, the clinicians agree—with near unanimity—that they would never go back to paper.

The sidebar account of the KP HealthConnect implementation in Kaiser Permanente's large Southern California region conveys many of the technical and human challenges as they played out in virtually every region, despite the larger scale of Southern California.

Slowing Down to Achieve Faster, More Effective Implementation

The rollout of KP HealthConnect in Kaiser Permanente's Southern California region was a complex undertaking involving twelve medical centers; more than 140 outpatient medical office buildings; and tens of thousands of doctors, nurses, and many other clinical and support personnel. Interfaces with hundreds of other systems had to be built; clinical departments from the entire region had to come together to determine common builds for the application and decide on common order sets; technical support and training personnel had to be hired and themselves trained; and elaborate schedules for each site and department required efficient deployment of limited resources. This was all background to the massive changes in workflow and culture required for a successful deployment.

The schedule was aggressive—first the business modules, then the outpatient clinical modules in rapid succession, one medical center at a time, and then the more complex inpatient modules in several phases involving clinical documentation, clerk order entry, and finally physician order entry. All this was to happen over a four-year timeframe.

The inevitable systems problems and implementation glitches surfaced. Clinical efficiency dropped, and workflows designed for paper records could not easily be adapted to a digital environment. Extra trainers were required. The ten-year program-wide cost estimate ballooned as these issues developed. The aggressive implementation schedule also created extreme stress on the core IT systems, forcing a six-month halt to the implementation schedule as our IT department scrambled to solve the problems.

Slowing down turned out to be the best thing that happened to Southern California. We took the time to solve many of the glitches in the system and to reconfigure workflows to better capitalize on the digital tool. We created training "sandboxes" for our physicians and other personnel that allowed them to familiarize themselves with the application and the changes in workflow required prior to going live. We leveraged expert users from one medical center to help others who were going live. Key physicians and other personnel from "downstream" facilities on the implementation queue were brought in to help and learn from sister facilities.

These and other changes enabled medical center productivity to come back more quickly and allowed for smoother and faster implementations.

Similar techniques were used for the inpatient system go-lives. We revamped the phased approach, enabling us to shave a year off the implementation schedule and ultimately saving over half a billion dollars off the peak ten-year cost estimates for the Southern California implementation and ongoing support. Even more important, a less costly, more efficient deployment enabled us to use the newly available information to create robust population and panel management tools that our doctors have leveraged to achieve incredible improvements in clinical outcomes for our members. Sometimes it is important to slow down before going fast.

—Ben Chu, MD, president, Kaiser Permanente-Southern California

Conclusion

By late 2005, all eight Kaiser Permanente regions had achieved successful, if incomplete, deployments, and the sharing of successful practices across regions was common. The deployment teams had begun attending the Epic Users' Group Meeting (UGM) each year, where Epic customers from many organizations shared experiences and lessons learned. Since the Kaiser Permanente collaborative build and implementation plan were new to the Epic community, Kaiser Permanente hosted a number of these UGM sessions, as well as its own users' conference.

At the August 2005 KP HealthConnect users' conference in Oakland, California, David Brailer, MD, then the national coordinator for Health Information Technology for the U.S. Department of Health and Human Services (HHS), delivered the keynote address. Brailer was appointed by President George W. Bush to help increase the use of information technology (IT) in health care and achieve the goal of providing every American with a personal electronic health record within ten years (by 2015). "If you don't know you're a leader, step back, breathe, and realize that you are a leader," Brailer told the crowd of more than five hundred physicians, nurses, business professionals, IT experts, operations managers, and senior leaders. "Cherish the work you're doing." He added that the federal government was watching Kaiser Permanente closely and learning from them as it developed its own ten-year health IT strategy. "This is a one-time chance to get in place the foundations," said Brailer. "Organizations like [Kaiser Permanente] are necessary to propel us into the far future." Brailer's inspiring speech offered critical reinforcement for the ongoing implementation work—a signal that the mission was greater than any single user, department, or region. The mission was about doing what was right for the nation's health care.

As noted, the collaborative build and implementation brought about and also enabled a cultural shift in the organization. Prior to the collaborative build, Kaiser Permanente was very much eight independent regions, each with its own leadership, strategic plans, and culture. While the intent of the collaborative build was to produce a common IT system, it did much more: it created a common organizational culture. Supported by technology, people made changes that had profound impacts on how they relate to one another and to their patients. The organization had shifted to a culture that valued collaboration, understood the power of coming together for a shared goal, and believed that implementing an enterprise-wide EHR was not only possible at Kaiser Permanente, it could be done best at Kaiser Permanente. The transformation in the culture and the changes that occurred bring to mind a popular quote from Henry Ford: "Coming together is a beginning; staying together is progress; and working together is success!"

Although the tools within KP HealthConnect are fully operational today, an important next step will be the sharing of electronic health records among regions. The Northern California and Southern California regions are currently working on a pilot to do this in early 2010. Other regions will follow. In the Colorado and Southern California regions, we are working with other organizations to share medical information for individual patients between different organizations. We believe these pilots will help further the coordination of care both inside and outside of Kaiser Permanente for all patients.

Lessons Learned

Although Kaiser Permanente has a unique structure, its experience of large-scale information technology implementation is relevant to complex health care organizations of all types and sizes. While other organizations may not have the same regional or national issues, every organization has internal variations in culture, structure, and processes—all of which must be overcome to make the best use of any IT system. Key lessons learned from the design and implementation of KP HealthConnect include the following:

- Leadership and sponsorship make a difference. Senior leaders must be engaged directly in the project work. Ideally, they should train on the system alongside staff and maintain a visible presence in the clinic during go-lives. Senior leaders can also help by eliminating or moving other key initiatives that could compete for resources.

- Involvement and ownership by business and operational leaders—not just IT people—are critical to success.
- Standardization and consistency must be balanced with the need for local modification. Local work process and IT system variations and different priorities may necessitate variation.
- Information technology is the "great magnifier" of broken processes. Operational issues must be addressed at the outset of the project or they will still be there later—and harder to resolve—once the system is implemented.
- When it comes time for users to start working with the new system, front-line supervisors are key to helping integrate the EHR into daily work. They know and are trusted by their staffs.
- Training should include all departments, not just clinical departments, and it should be user-centric rather than system-centric.
- Information technology systems drive massive change, and strategies to help people assimilate the change are essential.

CHAPTER THREE

PHYSICIAN LEADERSHIP AND ENGAGEMENT

By Andrew M. Wiesenthal, MD

Chapter Summary

This chapter looks at the three types of physician leaders who were critical to the success of the KP HealthConnect implementation—operational leaders, opinion leaders, and the technically adept. For a successful deployment, strong physician leadership in all aspects and phases of electronic health record selection, design, and implementation is an absolute requirement.

Introduction

One of the crucial components of a successful electronic health record (EHR) implementation is the effective engagement of clinicians in the entire process. In an integrated delivery system, the word *clinicians* assumes a broad meaning, incorporating physicians, nurses, pharmacy professionals, and many other licensed professionals. People in each of these categories were important to the success of Kaiser Permanente HealthConnect.

Andrew M. Wiesenthal, MD, SM, is an associate executive director of The Permanente Federation. He served as the Permanente medical groups' chief sponsor for the implementation of KP HealthConnect.

This chapter will deal explicitly with physicians, in order to increase the relevance of the lessons learned for delivery systems that may be less integrated than Kaiser Permanente.

Those of us in leadership positions who were ultimately accountable for the success of our project were familiar with the key role physicians play in clinical information technology. Our own organization had many positive and negative examples, and health care at large is no different. If key physicians are an active part of the process, you have an opportunity to succeed. If they are not, failure is nearly guaranteed.

This chapter will address a series of questions. Who are the key physicians, and how can they be identified and recruited to an implementation team? What additional training, if any, will they require? Once identified, what parts of the end-to-end project should they play a role in? What are their roles when they do participate—decision makers, subject-matter experts, leaders, evaluators? How should they be organized? How much time should they dedicate to the project? Should they be compensated for their involvement? Once initial implementation has occurred, what is their continuing role?

The Key Physicians

Key physicians fall into three "capability" groups—operational leaders, opinion leaders, and the technically adept. These groups are not mutually exclusive, yet it is rare to identify someone who has significant capability in all three areas. Since all three capabilities are needed for a project to succeed, more than one physician may have to participate, even on the smallest implementation teams.

Operational leaders are the doctors who are accountable for managing a group of people and a budget. In large medical groups like those at Kaiser Permanente, they lead departments or medical centers. Similarly, on hospital medical staffs or at academic medical centers, they are often the leaders of departments that are hospital-based. In certain ways, the physician who runs a small practice is an operational leader.

Opinion leaders are the doctors to whom the other doctors listen. They are judged to be good-to-excellent clinicians with a superior command of their practice lives, and other doctors model their behaviors and their decisions after them. If they declare publicly that they are prepared to take a certain action, they influence most of the other physicians in their affinity group to strongly consider doing the same. They are sometimes the operational leaders, but often they are not.

The definition of the technically adept physicians is self-evident. These are the doctors who know their way around computers. Many of them have been self-taught, but increasing numbers are university-trained computer scientists, graduates of fellowship training programs in clinical informatics, or both. If they have an opinion about a piece of hardware or software, other physicians will listen carefully, particularly if it is a negative opinion. If they are enthusiastic about a technical solution, other doctors often remain wary, dubious of their own abilities to master something that the technophile likes.

The good news is that these three types are not hard to find. The operational leaders are generally obvious—they are the ones with the titles and positions in a hierarchy. The opinion leaders manifest themselves in meetings, much like the old television advertisement for the brokerage firm E. F. Hutton—"when E. F. Hutton speaks, everyone listens." Once a group of doctors is repeatedly observed paying intense attention to one of their number, you have your opinion leader (nurses can often tell you who this is very quickly). The technically adept physicians are the easiest of all—once they know a project is under way, they will come to you.

Why are they all necessary? The operational leaders have to be on board because they often have a clear sense of what will and will not work from a practical standpoint in any clinical environment. If something is going to be hard to do, and EHR implementations are almost always hard to do, they are the ones who will have to make it work (or convince you that it has to be changed). If the opinion leaders commit to adopting a new EHR, the others are likely to follow. The technically adept can form a vital semantic and working bridge between the pure information technology professionals and the pure clinicians. When any of the myriad software configuration decisions is being made as a project progresses, these doctors with a foot in both worlds are a vital resource.

The approach to recruiting the key physicians also differs by their category. Time is perceived to be the most important ingredient by the operational leaders and the opinion leaders. They are fully occupied by their current work. If you want them to participate in a meaningful way in a complex, lengthy project, they cannot be expected to do so in the early mornings and late afternoons as an add-on or afterthought appended to full-time jobs. They have to be given dedicated time, very often half of their time, and, occasionally, all of their time, for the duration of the implementation. Someone has to assume responsibility for the portion of their administrative duties or practice that they give up, they have to be paid fairly for the time that they give, and they have to be provided with a smooth reintegration path into their former full-time jobs once the project is over, assuming that is what they want. The technically adept will often not express the need for time, because they are in love with the technology, but they need it just the same, and on the same terms.

Identifying and recruiting the key physicians played out for KP HealthConnect along the lines described above. The technically adept either came forward quickly or were already involved in existing, related EHR projects. We had to entice the operational leaders and the opinion leaders, and we accomplished that with two key elements of our overall strategy—setting a vision and involvement in the collaborative build—that have been described in previous chapters. Participation in vendor selection was also an important component of engaging all three groups. Finally, all were thoroughly involved in the development and maintenance of clinical content, which will be addressed later in this chapter.

Involving Physicians in Creating the Blue Sky Vision

In the first phase of the Blue Sky visioning process (described in Chapter One), we engaged all three types of physicians. Senior operational leaders, opinion leaders, and technical adepts all participated in developing a common understanding of the medium-term future of health care in the United States. They helped create the vision in 2003, literally acting it out, and they had the opportunity to listen to the opinions of others from both inside and outside the organization as we built a description of the health care ideal for 2015.

The second phase was intentionally devoted exclusively to operational leaders, both physicians and nonphysicians. We purposely recruited an entirely new set of the latter, nearly two dozen of them, for this phase. They were asked to create the practical steps connecting our current state (in 2003) with the ideal state of 2015, with a particular focus on how technology, and EHRs in particular, could help us transform our organization to meet the vision.

The process was exciting for all participants, and all of them, including the involved physicians, grasped the ideas and ultimately spread them to thousands of colleagues by word of mouth, by publication in *The Permanente Journal* (the quarterly journal of the Permanente medical groups, distributed to all Permanente physicians), and by formal presentation. It is not possible to overestimate the importance of the clarity of this vision and the extent of its dissemination. We knew what the goal was: the transformation of the health care delivery system to a new ideal state. We knew what the steps on the road to that new ideal state were. Finally, we knew that an EHR was a critical enabler for many of those steps, and, even more important, that the deployment of the EHR was not the goal—system transformation was.

To cynics, all of this may sound like so much fluff. Perhaps it was, but there is no doubt that it captured the imaginations of scores of physician leaders, who then captured scores more. The constancy of purpose engendered by the Blue Sky Vision helped senior physician leaders make difficult decisions and helped the entire body of physicians remember why they were doing what they were doing when the deployment of the EHR got tough. And it did get tough.

Vendor Selection

Just as physician leaders played a key role in establishing the vision, they also occupied a prominent place as we selected our vendor. They established what we aimed to achieve, and they were part of a large group of individuals charged with selecting a means to that end—the software we would use.

First, they helped establish an important set of ground rules, chief among which was that we strongly preferred an integrated suite of software. We wanted documentation tools, order entry, results reporting, decision support, registration and scheduling, and billing and other business functionality, all built from the start to work together across the continuum of care. We were not interested in identifying the best of each category of software and then integrating all of that independently developed code. We wanted things that were designed up front to work together, even if it meant selecting software in which some individual components were not the best in their class.

The physician leaders then engaged in demonstrations, technical and functional assessments, and site visits to vendors and other health systems, and finally participated directly in formulating a recommendation. They achieved extraordinary consensus around our ultimate selection, software from Epic Systems, Inc., even when some individuals openly acknowledged that, for their special needs, they preferred software from another vendor. Participation with true influence in this part of our process turned these physicians into "owners" of the decision, people who felt accountable both for explaining the decision to their colleagues and making sure that the ensuing implementation project would succeed. They even participated extensively in selecting the name of our project: KP HealthConnect. While almost none of them reported to me in a strictly hierarchical sense, it was this phase of our work together that legitimized me as a convener, coordinator, decision maker, and supporter of their efforts—the national senior executive sponsor for the Permanente medical group physicians (the Permanente side of Kaiser Permanente).

Physician Leader Training

All of the participating physicians, in each of the three categories, needed training once vendor selection was concluded. All of them needed to learn the applications we were licensing as an end-user would learn about them. Beyond that (and that was substantial, given that there were hundreds of them), their training requirements diverged. The opinion leaders needed to learn about the way in which the functionality was going to affect the practices and workflows for themselves and their peers. What was going to be good or easy about adopting these tools? What was going to be difficult? Where were the usability barriers that we would have to address or at least openly acknowledge?

The operational leaders needed to be made aware of these answers, too. They also needed to understand how they could use the functionality to drive the organization toward the Blue Sky Vision and toward the more formal and concrete business case goals we had set as milestones on the path to that vision. What could documentation tools achieve for us? What could we do with the decision support tools embedded with the software? How would it help us meet regulatory requirements, reporting requirements, and revenue capture requirements? In short, how would we be able to use it to transform the process of care delivery, leveraging our highly integrated model?

Finally, our "techies" needed training on the "dark side" of the application. How did the data model work? What were the configuration decisions that could be made, and what tools were available to execute those decisions? What were all of the different clinical content tools at our disposal, and how were they designed?

Once all of this was accomplished, all of them needed to learn how to collaborate iteratively among themselves and with many other professionals. This collaboration (our "collaborative build" discussed in Chapter Two) allowed us to structure the data model and make the configuration decisions that would support care delivery transformation by improving physician effectiveness, thus enabling delivery of the Blue Sky Vision. This was the health information technology version of the "house that Jack built." Providing this training further strengthened the sense of ownership for all of these physicians, and it created a large cohort of individuals who were capable of training their colleagues to use the system. Further, they could explain to their colleagues how and why configuration decisions were made the way they were.

Clinical Content

Particular attention must be paid to the role these three groups of clinicians played in the development of clinical content for the system. Clinical content is anything that contributes to guiding the ways in which physicians document and order. Broadly speaking, clinical content, in all its forms, is equivalent to decision support. Many clinicians may think of decision support in a narrow sense—alerts that pop up to prevent errors or to remind users to execute certain tasks. But EHR technology allows for a much more expansive range of ways to support making the right thing the easiest thing to do. Examples range from lists of order types for specific specialties, to clusters of orders focused on specific clinical problems, to "forms" to document with, to alerts to guide decisions or avoid errors, and more. Physicians must be involved in identifying and developing all such content.

Closing the "quality chasm"—a crucial element driving the business case for the use of EHRs—can be achieved only when content is designed to encourage care that is based on the best available evidence and to discourage care that is not. The content in EHRs, if well designed, can make the right thing the easiest thing to do. If poorly designed, it can render the EHR close to useless. In order to achieve the former and minimize the risk of the latter, physicians have to design the content.

As one might expect, all three groups had to participate in content design. Operational leaders knew the clinical objectives of the practice—they kept design focused on what mattered most. Opinion leaders knew what would work best for doctors and what they were likely to accept (and what changes in workflow they were willing to lead those other doctors through). The technically adept knew how to use the design tools in the software to greatest effect—which tools to use, how suitable they were to the desired task, and how to minimize errors in their use.

The process of design was iterative, and the initial content produced, especially when the physicians had little or no actual experience using the software to do their work, was often inadequate to downright bad. Here, the opinion leaders were most valuable, because they sold the initial content as a work-in-progress that was expected to need substantial refinement based on user feedback. The operational leaders compensated for initially inadequate content (as well as the learning curve for the software functionality itself) by expecting physicians and nurses to be inefficient as the software was first being implemented and cutting back on workloads (we reduced work expectations by 50 percent for a couple of weeks and then gradually returned to 100 percent). They planned "backfill" for that inefficiency so that service to Kaiser Permanente members was never compromised. The technical adepts were organized to support rapid turnaround of modifications as feedback was received.

This entire process ultimately needed to be made permanent, because new content will always be needed, old content will always need updating, and new software functionality will routinely enable new approaches to old problems.

Clinicians Won't Necessarily Be Faster, But They Should Be Better

It has often been assumed that unless the EHR made the clinician "faster" it would not be accepted. But one of our key learnings in implementing KP HealthConnect's precursor, the Epic-based ambulatory EHR in Kaiser Permanente's Northwest region, is that clinicians are initially slower after EHR implementation. Over time, some clinicians will become faster than they were before, but many will remain slower. But even the slower clinicians recognize the value of information technology—and given the choice, would not want to return to the pre-EHR days. Our theory is that clinicians are able to trade off their own increased workload against the improvement in care and professional satisfaction that they see with the use of the EHR. With changes in the paradigm of care delivery that the EHR enables, even the "slower" physicians will be more efficient in their overall care of a given population of members.

—Homer Chin, MD, Kaiser Permanente-Northwest

Content development is something that a large medical group, or, in our case, a group of medical groups, can take on with little to no external help. Small practices will not have the resources to do this work. One alternative is to purchase content.

There are vendors that sell and maintain content for at least some specialties, but not all. Specialty societies and academic medical centers will likely fill this void as standard approaches to the incorporation of independently developed content into EHR software become available (they are not yet). In addition, the Regional Health Information Technology Extension Centers provided for in the 2009 federal stimulus legislation could also play a role. Right now, most physicians in small practices are probably stuck with whatever content their EHR software vendor supplies, unless they choose to devote substantial amounts of additional time to developing their own.

In the case of the Permanente medical groups, we relied extensively on our internal Care Management Institute (CMI) for much of the crucial evidence analysis, guideline development, and seed ideas and forms for much of our content. The CMI is a joint venture of the Kaiser Foundation Health Plan and the Permanente Medical Groups, founded in 1997 expressly to perform these functions, and it has since developed nation-leading strategies and formats to support the delivery of excellent, evidence-based care.

Implementation

All of the preceding is a prelude to implementing the software itself. In this stage, which seems superficially to be a mostly technical exercise, physician leadership and engagement were more important than ever. Planning every element of implementation—end user training, the timing and sequencing of the different go-lives (departments, facilities, and so on), the nature of support as the go-lives occurred—was led by and managed by physicians. Here the operational leaders had the primary role, with the opinion leaders often acting as primary communicators and the technical adepts doing rapid turnaround reconfiguration and content redesign as problems were identified.

At this juncture, we identified a fourth category of physician useful to us, because our roll-out, simply due to our size, was going to occur over a period of at least several weeks, if not months to years, depending on the operating region. These were our "superusers." They were physicians who just "got it," in terms of using the software to work efficiently in their specialty. They were sometimes also technical adepts, but more often they were a new addition to the team. They quickly were freed temporarily of practice responsibilities and mobilized to provide "at the elbow" support for other physicians in their specialty as the latter began to use the software. The following approach summarizes the nature of the help they gave: "When I want to do what you are trying to do, here is how I do it." This type of support turned out to be the most effective training tool at our disposal, and we ultimately reduced pre-go-live didactic or computer-based training and amplified the use of superusers whenever possible, to good effect. Most of our superusers have returned to full-time practice, though some have become permanent members of the regional support teams.

Assessing Physician Readiness

There are many key factors in the successful implementation of an EHR. Because the tool's ultimate success depends so heavily on how front-line physicians use it, it is imperative that physicians understand the change, are clear about what is expected of them (for example, all physicians will use the EHR), and are assured that the organization will do its part to position them for success. Three critical success factors in our EHR implementation in Kaiser Permanente's Georgia region were leadership engagement and visibility, a physician-focused communication plan, and the comprehensive readiness assessment we conducted of physicians and staff.

The objective of the readiness assessment was to evaluate and ensure the readiness of all clinicians, departments, teams, and staff for the implementation of the EHR. We developed a tool that allowed us to assess overall skills and knowledge, attitude and motivation, teamwork/working relationships, work processes and conditions, leadership, comfort with use of automated systems, and basic computer skills. Our findings allowed us to create a comprehensive plan that addressed needs at the individual, department, and team level, as appropriate. Facilitators were assigned to insure implementation of the plan and to follow the progress of individuals, teams, and departments. Our motto was to assure that "no doc was left behind."

The comprehensive attention to physician preparation not only allowed us to help our physicians prepare for the change but bought us a great deal of good will at a time of disruptive transformation in our organization.

—Debra Carlton, MD, Kaiser Permanente-Georgia

Post-Implementation

It is important to note that, in certain ways, implementation has never ended and probably never will. We are always trying to use the tools better, something we call optimization, and we expect routinely to upgrade the software as the vendor improves the technical performance of the software and adds functionality we value. The competencies our three categories of physicians have acquired have become permanently needed. Our operational leaders will always need to understand the software and how it can be used to improve operations and reach our clinical goals. Our opinion leaders will always be touchstones for usability and effective workflow design, and our technical adepts will always be bridging between their understanding of how the software works and their understanding of how clinical practice works.

Initial and Ongoing Roles

In our experience, then, physicians have a special role in the development of the clinical vision, elaborating what the ideal clinical future ought to be for the organization. They are decision makers, certainly addressing the question of what software will be licensed to support that vision. They have to be planners, laying out the strategy and tactics for deployment of the software for the physician practices. They have to be subject-matter experts, particularly as it pertains to the development and use of clinical content within the software. They have to iteratively and constantly evaluate the use and effectiveness of the software, participating in refining or changing decisions made during the initial software build. Finally, and most important, they have to lead the clinical aspects of the project. While information technologists—software and hardware engineers—are fundamental to the success of any EHR implementation, they are necessary but definitely not sufficient if that implementation is to be successful. Physicians have to be visible and actual leaders along with other key clinical and operational leaders.

Kaiser Permanente uses a model project structure that involves executive sponsorship, a steering committee, and dedicated project teams. Executive sponsors are senior leaders who can make final decisions, command resources, and remove barriers to success. Steering committee members are dedicated to the acceptance and oversight of a detailed project plan, keeping the project on time and on budget by addressing problems that the project team encounters or escalating those problems to the executive sponsors if they cannot resolve them. The project team develops the project plan and executes the day-to-day tactics inherent in delivering on the plan. Nationally, there were two executive sponsors for KP HealthConnect, including myself as the senior physician leader. Our national steering committee comprised senior operational leaders from around our organization, more than half of whom were physician executives, and the national project team had both physician and nonphysician members, the former being mostly technically adept physicians. This structure and composition was replicated in each of our eight operating regions, with physicians just as prominently involved at that level. In the end, hundreds of physicians were involved if we account for all of the superusers as part of the regional project teams.

All of this involvement was not an afterthought. It was felt to be necessary for physicians to have dedicated, compensated time to devote to the work. In the case of physician project team leaders, this was often full-time work for several years. Most others were part time, generally 50 percent, also for several years. While the sizes of our national and regional teams have been reduced substantially as initial implementation has been completed, we still maintain both a national team and regional teams, generally about a quarter of their peak sizes, with a proportional level of permanent physician involvement. We expect to permanently maintain these teams in some form.

Conclusion and Lessons Learned

It is important to remind the reader that this chapter has been devoted to describing the initial and ongoing roles of physicians in KP HealthConnect. Many other types of clinicians, notably nurses, pharmacy professionals, laboratory technicians, and scores of others were vital in every aspect of this work. Physician engagement is essential and absolutely necessary, but certainly not sufficient.

Still, physician engagement was clearly at the very heart of our project, and a vital element in its success. Without our operational leaders, opinion leaders, and technically adept physicians, we would have accomplished little to nothing, and we certainly could not have deployed KP HealthConnect in an organization of our size in the relatively short time that it took. What are our lessons learned in the area of physician engagement?

- Identify, support, and involve vital physician leaders in every category—opinion leaders, operational leaders, and technical adepts;
- Give physician leaders the time, the training, and the resources to succeed;
- Involve them in a meaningful way in every step of the process—setting the vision, communicating the vision, selecting the vendor, configuring the software, developing clinical content, training end users, deploying the software, and optimizing the use of the system after initial deployment; and
- Permanently support a core of engaged physicians of each type to accomplish continuing transformation.

CHAPTER FOUR

NURSING LEADERSHIP AND IMPACT

By Marilyn P. Chow, RN, DNSc, and Valerie Fong, RN

Chapter Summary

This chapter examines the critical role of nursing leaders in the successful implementation of an electronic health record (EHR), especially in the inpatient, or hospital, setting. As in the case of the outpatient EHR implementation, nurses collaborated across Kaiser Permanente's eight regions to help design, build, and validate tools for standardized documentation of patient care and innovative, evidence-based approaches to quality improvement.

Introduction

If there is any group in health care, besides physicians, that knows the limitations, inefficiencies, and dangers in paper medical records, it is nurses.

Kaiser Permanente employs more than 40,000 nurses across the country, and we welcomed the opportunity to be involved in this large-scale transformation from a paper to an electronic world, a change that we believed would improve patient care.

Marilyn P. Chow, RN, DNSc, is Kaiser Permanente's vice president of National Patient Care Services; Valerie Fong, RN, MS, is senior manager of Care Delivery Transitions.

While quality care has always been foundational in our organization, it was clear to us that Kaiser Permanente HealthConnect would not only facilitate improved clinical documentation to support improved care but also help us gain a truer understanding of what constitutes best nursing practice.

The most important aspect of our strategic vision for nursing was to enable nurses to consistently deliver the best and most reliable care across all care settings. KP HealthConnect would facilitate our ability to compare "like" information across practice settings, thereby helping to determine the best ways to deliver care while hastening the development of organization-wide nursing standards that could be implemented at the local and national levels. It would lead to standardization for electronically recording patient information, enabling more predictive tracking of how nursing can best contribute to successful patient outcomes.

Initially, Kaiser Permanente's implementation of the EHR focused primarily on physician workflow and processes in the outpatient setting. Given the higher visibility of nurse contributions in the care of hospitalized patients, our nursing vision focused on implementing the inpatient EHR, with greater emphasis on nursing governance and on creating standardized content and work procedures. This chapter focuses on the lessons learned from our experiences in establishing a collaborative or common build for nursing in our thirty-six hospitals across the country—a collaboration that ultimately produced content with the same look, definition, and meaning.

Involving Nurses from the Outset

On our journey from paper medical records to electronic records, nurses were included from the outset not only in vendor selection but, more important, in the planning process—we helped design, build, and validate standards for gathering, organizing, and displaying patient information on the computer system.

Early on, we knew a well-designed EHR was critical to support the practice and delivery of clinical nursing care. We wanted a robust clinical system that was intuitive for nursing staff and that would drive improvements in patient care outcomes and nursing clinical practices. It was also essential to have common nursing documentation content, including the same look, same context, same flow—content that would be the same at all Kaiser Permanente nursing facilities.

At the highest level, our vision was to establish common standards, goals, and objectives for nurses across the organization, a uniformity that always reflected best care practices. Nursing leadership at all levels was essential to the success of this vision.

To achieve this success, however, we needed to address a major nursing frustration—more time with paper than with patients. The results of a 2008 Kaiser Permanente and Ascension Health national time-and-motion study validated this frustration in finding that a typical medical-surgical nurse spent an average of 35.3 percent of a ten-hour shift on clinical documentation (recording patient care activities, medication information, and ongoing health status) (Hendrich and others, 2008). Economist David Cutler cited this study in his annual cost estimate of health care documentation, which he calculated at an astonishing $50 billion (Cutler, 2009).

Our challenge, then, was to design an electronic documentation system for nurses that captured vital patient information as part of their work while minimizing their documentation burden. The documentation also needed to incorporate increasing quality measurement requirements and accreditation regulations of oversight agencies.

Improving Patient Safety with Electronic Documentation

The Institute of Medicine report, *Keeping Patients Safe: Transforming the Work Environment of Nurses* (Institute of Medicine, 2004), examined patient safety from intersecting perspectives: from that of the work environment, where patient care is delivered, and from the perspective of nursing work practice characteristics, since nurses represent the largest component of the health care workforce. The report presented evidence about the critical nursing role in surveillance and interception of medical errors before they adversely affect patients, and it examined nurses' documentation burden. It concluded that computer technology is an effective means of preventing medical errors, assuming systems are carefully designed to incorporate workflows with appropriate software functionality.

Toward that end, through a conference grant from the Robert Wood Johnson Foundation, Kaiser Permanente collaborated with our vendor Epic's Nursing Advisory Council, a group of nursing leaders from health care organizations that were using the Epic system. They sought to understand better how to design and use the EHR to deliver safe patient care, particularly in terms of capturing nursing performance measures such as documentation of patient care activities and medication administration.

During the design phase, KP HealthConnect needed to facilitate the nurse's ability to compare "like" information across practice settings, thereby promoting quality care. This information included things as basic as medical terminology, and so we eliminated the use of confusing but nonfunctional brand names; thus, "indwelling urinary catheter" replaced "Foley catheter," and "hydrophilic polyurethane" replaced "Tegaderm." This clarified the use of supplies and materials, devices, and drugs, and eventually standardized identification, tracking, and evaluation by function, not brand name. We similarly created standard data definitions for describing a patient's intravenous (IV) line along a continuum of "pain," "numbness," "tingling," and "discoloration"—a standard and defined range that every nurse would use for documentation regardless of patient type, age, or location.

We also envisioned organization-wide standardization of nursing clinical content that would eventually lead to the identification of successful patient outcomes related to the contribution of nurses. For example, analysis of preliminary data gathered through KP HealthConnect on pressure ulcers shows strong evidence that a patient's continence and prior ability to move are statistically associated with his or her likelihood of developing these ulcers. Currently, we are using the data to develop a predictive model for risk of pressure ulcers that will help nurses prevent them. Overall efforts to standardize the terminology used in KP HealthConnect by nurses have, in effect, already begun to improve care and increase efficiencies.

Developing Nursing Leadership

Initially, the collaborative design of nursing clinical content to be used in KP Health-Connect was largely driven by the KP HealthConnect national and regional teams. These teams were responsible for the overall project, with the help of subject matter experts from each of the four Kaiser Permanente regions that owned hospitals (Hawaii, Northwest, Northern California, and Southern California). However, major nursing decisions were left to a subset of Kaiser Permanente's Inter-regional Nursing Council (INC), the body that sets the strategic direction for nursing practice across the organization's care continuum. INC members include nursing operations leaders from all eight Kaiser Permanente regions and across all care settings (ambulatory, advice centers, hospitals, and home health), representatives of nursing labor unions that are part of the Kaiser Permanente Labor Management Partnership (LMP), and the organization's national leaders of quality, safety, and compliance.

In early 2004, the INC envisioned a clinical information system that must (1) promote evidence-based practice, (2) support a professional practice framework, and (3) enable point-of-care documentation. Central to the vision was the need to standardize nursing practice and reduce variation. With the development of a flow sheet to capture patient admission and shift assessment data, the number of documentation fields was decreased by eliminating assessment descriptors that either were not used by all regions or added only minimal information. For example, the twenty paper record fields for describing basic neurological findings were reduced to four in the electronic record, consistent across all regions.

Through this process of review and consensus, we first created a standard content model for use for all adult medical-surgical patients, the vast majority of hospitalizations. This generalist content served as the foundation for the design and build for other domains and specialties such as critical care and pediatrics.

The next step was to vet the content with operational teams at the regional level. Key criteria were developed to evaluate requests for changes to the standard content: (1) patient safety, (2) legal and compliance requirements, (3) clinical appropriateness,

(4) evidence-based nursing review, and 5) technical impact. The number of change requests grew to 1,200, with the largest percentage having patient safety listed as the rationale, but most change requests also reflected attempts to retain the historical way of practicing. This rash of change requests helped us realize the need for greater involvement from front-line nursing.

By early 2005, the INC had established an Inter-regional Nursing Governance Group (INGG) to address this need for collaboration, clear communication, and ownership of the transition from paper to the EHR by regional nursing leadership. The INGG provided operational oversight and strategic direction from nursing operations, and it continues to serve as the accountable decision-making governance group with representation from all nursing labor unions for the inpatient nursing build. Still, the initial challenge was daunting. Nothing of this magnitude, much less learning how to collaborate across regions, had ever been attempted for nursing at Kaiser Permanente.

Several initial INGG meetings lasted over ten hours each, during which the entire list of 1,200 change requests was reviewed and decided on. This huge time commitment for group members helped to forge valuable relationships and build trust and commitment. The INGG's comprehensive collaboration between nursing operations, KP HealthConnect teams, and labor union partners was something we would call upon often.

Working Collaboratively

Prior to KP HealthConnect, each of our four regions with hospitals, and even the medical centers within those regions, had differing practices of nursing documentation and clinical care. For example, all medical-surgical departments in the thirteen medical centers in our Southern California region were using the same Adult Admission Assessment form, but the twenty-one medical centers in our Northern California region were using more than twelve variations of the same paper forms. Most of these intra-regional and inter-regional variations were related to facility infrastructure, hospital work procedures, and patient care dynamics, all of which varied in addition with local culture and leadership style. While the decision to have one nursing collaborative build was an easy one, the journey toward making this a reality was much more complicated.

At the beginning of the nursing content design process, we developed an assessment documentation strategy. Central to this strategy was decreasing the amount of time a nurse would spend with documentation, decreasing the time spent on defining assessment types, and defining "normal" patient assessment criteria. Similar reductions related to use of "general" versus "complex" flow sheet rows and expectations for completing flow sheets.

Nothing was simple. Collaborative discussion revealed that even nursing leaders had different interpretations of assessment types. Likewise, discussions and agreements on the use of standardized references and assessment tools for skin risk, pain, and sedation were very lengthy but necessary steps in establishing and fostering inter-regional rapport and networking.

As part of this process, the INGG carefully reviewed the nursing practices in each region and adopted them where appropriate. For example, our Northwest region used a questionnaire, CAGE, as a standard tool to identify risk of alcoholism as part of its routine admission assessment. The other regions were unfamiliar with the tool but eventually agreed to incorporate it into KP HealthConnect. And when conflicts arose related to different state law requirements, we chose the default of incorporating the more stringent rules that would push nursing practices to the highest level.

Another successful INGG collaborative decision involved creating a set of standard patient care goals that were to be applied to any patient admitted to the hospital regardless of location in the hospital or diagnosis. The goals were basic: the patient is safe, comfortable, knows what to expect from the hospital stay, and participates with care givers in the development of his or her treatment plan. Creating these basic goals brought a greater sense of cohesiveness to the group and eventually increased ownership of the transition from paper to electronic records. The INGG decisions were recorded and the rationale was captured. The documented rationale would later be used to help support the regional leaders in presenting the reasoning behind the changes to their front-line nurses.

A benefit was seen immediately when nurses at the Southern California region's first facility to go live wanted to add their own changes to the content. The regional nursing operations executive and KP HealthConnect partner stood firm in communicating that there would be only "one common build" to be shared across all of the individual facilities in the region. It represented a significant culture change for nursing leaders to feel empowered to uphold the "one build" mantra, and it resulted in fewer requests for changes to nursing content in subsequent Southern California go-lives. What's more, subsequent change requests were of high quality and high value. This became a key lesson for other regions, as participants saw how much strong leadership behavior modeling and sponsorship during the collaborative build aided the transformation.

Culture change in any hospital setting is an acknowledged nursing leadership challenge. Managing all the necessary steps involved in a large-scale, clinical transformation and establishing national standardization by incorporating evidence-based content was daunting, yet vital to our ability as an organization to reach measurable results in quality care. The INGG members promoted nurse awareness and involvement and continue to do that as they have successfully executed the adoption and integration of innovative workflows with content and functionality in KP HealthConnect.

Preparing Nursing Leaders for the EHR

Early on, nursing leaders needed to recognize that moving to an EHR did not mean copying current paper forms and recreating them in electronic form. Preparing nursing leaders for the digital age cannot be underestimated. Although most nurse managers acknowledged that things would change during the transition, few recognized that their everyday work as leaders would also change.

Entering the Digital Age of Nursing

Anecdotal observation following the inpatient EHR implementation revealed that implementations proceeded more smoothly among nursing staff whose managers and leaders embraced computer technology. Even in our very connected and fast-paced world, it cannot be assumed that all nursing leaders are "tech savvy," given that the average age of nurses in 2009 was forty-eight years, and nurse leaders are apt to be older. So it is natural to assume that a fair number of the currently practicing nursing population has never had formal computer education and is likely to be wary, at least, of something as daunting as a complex EHR implementation.

Nurse managers who embraced computer technology and exhibited enthusiasm about the implementation in their communications and interactions with staff members elicited positive responses from their staffs and experienced successful adoption of the technology after go-live. Conversely, nursing units where the manager was unfamiliar with computer technology or wary of it had a much more difficult transition, and the difficulties and negative attitudes about the EHR persisted well past the go-live. The attitude of nursing leaders was central to success.

Clearly, before embarking on an EHR project, organizations should prepare nursing leaders to move into the digital age by providing basic keyboarding and computer skills courses and teaching nurse managers how to use the features of a computer operating system, a word processing program, and presentation software. Last, all managers and staff nurses should be given access to and required to use a hospital e-mail system for communication. These may sound like simple ideas, but for the large population of mature nurses who have had very little exposure to computers, they could go a long way toward ensuring a successful EHR adoption.

— Julie Vilardi RN, MS, executive director, Kaiser Permanente Clinical Applications Group

To prepare themselves and their staffs for the change, nursing leaders, managers, and assistant managers received special training. Bettianne Wiessler, the nursing leader for the inpatient KP HealthConnect implementation in the twenty-one-hospital Northern California region, related her team's experience in persuading hospital nurse leaders to "own" the transition. As Wiessler told us,

Our approach consisted of providing hospital leaders, managers, and assistant managers with instructions on how to lead change in their hospitals through manager readiness classes, manager tools for preparing staff, key leadership messages regarding strategic hospital outcome goals, and mandating appropriate EHR training for leading nurses. Training included specific tools within the EHR for executives, managers, educators, clinical nurse specialists, and quality and infection control nurses. These classes focused on how to use specific tools for overseeing hospital operations and patient care delivery. Training for front-line staff nurses focused on how to deliver care using the EHR.

Nursing leaders and managers were taught how to log in every day to use revealing real-time and retrospective reports to oversee hospital operations and the delivery of care. Real-time reports provide immediate feedback to nurses on patient safety, regulatory and Joint Commission standards, core measures, and compliance documentation. A manager's ability to use these reports to monitor and respond while patients are in the hospital proved invaluable. Retrospective reports, which are used to trend performance over time, are critical in the initial roll-out to monitor staff compliance to meet target goals. Moreover, the ability to handle unannounced surveyors, such as the Joint Commission survey, was a key focus for review, as we needed to ensure that front-line staff had the confidence to navigate in the EHR to access key information.

Creating Nurse Champions

Another example of successful change management was the creation of nurse champions. These nurses not only assisted with the overall implementation of KP Health-Connect at the facility level but also led the overall cultural transformation with front-line staff.

Curtis N. Dikes, Kaiser Permanente's national director of clinical informatics technology integration, told us,

As the inpatient implementation ramped up for KP HealthConnect, responsibilities mounted on the regional nursing executives, who, given normal operations demands, had insufficient bandwidth for this complicated process. They needed informatics support to understand the implications of programming decisions, process changes, and then to recommend timelines for their medical centers. The regional clinical systems department supplied this support, but there were too many individual medical-center-level decisions to track in addition to addressing national and regional design and implementation needs. To relieve this burden, we created a new dedicated and paid position of nurse champion at the medical-center level, someone who could provide onsite support with an eye to local needs and was able to work with site implementation teams needing critical input. The nurse champions assisted with the preparation, training, implementation, and overall culture transformation. After implementation, the champion role was retained to work with KP HealthConnect optimization and improvement efforts on an ongoing basis.

Practice Change Innovations

The KP HealthConnect implementation process supported other key nursing practice changes. One of the earliest examples of this collaborative effort was the development of Nurse Knowledge Exchange (NKE), a standardized process developed with the assistance of IDEO, an innovation and design consultant, for shift change between the arriving and departing nurses. When our nurses first gathered to design the nursing clinical content for KP HealthConnect, they were asked, "What processes in your hospitals do you find challenging?" The top two responses were nurse communications at shift change and bed management. Before NKE, patients described the hospital floor during shift change as a "ghost town," since nurses would exchange information or shift reports behind the closed doors of a conference room or staff lounge. One component of NKE includes a standardized data template that serves as the key communication tool, assisting the departing nurse in preparing patient information for the shift change. The departing nurse conveys this information to the arriving nurse at the patient's bedside, and key information such as diet and expected hospital tests are also written on a whiteboard in the patient's room. This standardized process also ensures patient awareness of their status and ensures accurate expectations for their care. During the NKE pilot phase, we found that the time an arriving nurse spent preparing to see patients was reduced by 50 to 75 percent. Thus, NKE eliminated the "ghost town" effect—and patients felt more involved in their care. The standardized data template is now embedded in KP HealthConnect, ensuring that accurate, consistent information is available on each patient no matter who is delivering the care.

Medication Administration

Another valuable innovative practice change based on both high-tech and low-tech solutions involved a new approach to medication administration. With the help of our internal innovation consultants who had learned IDEO design approaches, KP MedRite was established to standardize and enhance the process of giving patients their medications. The national time and motion study referenced earlier found that nearly 20 percent of a nurse's work time (an average of 17.2 percent) was spent administering medication. We knew that dispensing medications and tracking them was a major patient safety issue that could be improved with KP HealthConnect and related process changes.

Before KP MedRite, nurses had described the many distractions that prevented them from feeling safe about medication administration. In fact, we documented that, on average, a nurse had at least one interruption by another staff member during the course of administering medication. With the EHR as a foundation, front-line staff designed a process that capitalized on KP HealthConnect functionality, integrated additional technology, and redesigned the workflow to be consistent throughout inpatient units.

To combat the interruption problem, nurses began wearing a brightly colored sash or vest while administering medications so their colleagues would know they should not be interrupted. Noninterrupt or sacred zones were also marked off around the medication dispensing machine. On the technology side, our Northern California region took the lead in using barcode scanning technology for medication administration, as described in the sidebar. These innovations resulted in a 50 percent reduction in the number of staff interruptions during medication and an 18 percent increase in the on-time administering of medications in our test sites. These innovations are being shared with other health care providers to benefit patients outside of Kaiser Permanente.

Barcode Medication Administration

In our Northern California hospitals, we implemented barcode medication administration (BCMA) as part of an EHR "Big Bang" (implementing all applications in all clinical units, all the same day). The technology includes a unique identifier (barcode) on the patient's wristband as well as barcodes on every dose of medication and IV solution. We utilized barcode scanners mounted on wireless mobile carts to enable medication administration at the patient's bedside. The nursing workflow involves scanning the patient's wristband to check patient identification and open the patient's electronic medication administration record in KP HealthConnect. This ensures we have the right patient. The nurse reviews medications due on the record and then scans each medication, verifying the right medication, right dose, right route, and right time.

The effectiveness of a BCMA safety system cannot rely on technology alone. Many factors must be solidly embedded to create and maintain a culture of safety. They include

- *Leadership Expectations:* The nursing leadership must prioritize BCMA as a required workflow for every medication administered.
- *Organizational Standards:* Nursing leadership set a standard of 5 percent or less overrides (bypassing the barcoding process), which became a major goal for every medical center.
- *Nurse Competency:* Nurses need to practice BCMA with actual patient wristbands and real medication barcodes in a safe "play" environment prior to use on patients. Competency documentation of each nurse prior to go-live is a key metric.

- *Reports:* During the first few weeks after go-live, daily reports of medication over-rides by facility, clinical area, and nurse allow for immediate feedback to nurses who create workarounds unless closely monitored. After achieving the goal of 5 percent or fewer overrides, monthly reports assist nurse managers in sustaining the correct workflows to prevent medication errors.
- *Feedback and Reward Mechanisms:* Providing simple but positive feedback to individual nurses who demonstrated correct and consistent BCMA workflows was an easy and effective success strategy.

— Ann O'Brien RN, MSN, director of Clinical Informatics, Kaiser Permanente-Northern California

Staff Satisfaction and Engagement

Despite such innovations, the transition from paper to electronic documentation is still immensely challenging for the front-line staff, as noted by Ziporah Watt, an intensive care unit staff nurse at Southern California's Riverside Medical Center:

The myth that "computer charting" is quick, easy, and time-saving was dispelled in the first KP HealthConnect training class I attended. The information imparted was overwhelming. It was quickly apparent that learning to use the system would be a long process and that these new skills would take time to hone. When we started using the system, it was a paradigm shift for everyone to be able to care for patients with much more information available to us than we were accustomed to on the paper record. The change affected my workflow, patient care delivery habits, and how I communicated with others. It also became clear that many workflows needed to be improved, which led to some significant efficiency gains.

Having experienced KP HealthConnect for some months, it is easy to see that the system instills good habits in nurses: documentation is more thorough while communication and referrals are stronger. But despite the wealth of information that KP HealthConnect brings to my fingertips, it is still important that we talk frequently and openly with one another to ensure high-quality care.

Conclusion and Lessons Learned

What we learned from the inpatient EHR processes reinforces the value of nursing in the ambulatory setting of medical offices. The system promotes lateral integration, while building capacity for evidence-based patient care practices and outcomes at the point of care. But without personal, effective, cross-functional relationships, innovation and optimization of ambulatory nursing care will not occur.

The transformation from paper to KP HealthConnect has required that we remain open to exploring new ways of doing things. During our journey, we have dealt with significant ambiguity and uncertainty. It is easy to forget about the many long days that the INGG spent solidifying the collaborative governance processes and the struggles of creating something from nothing—from "analysis paralysis" to tough decision making. Many disagreements resulted from poor communication among diverse stakeholders. But the result was that we have built effective, diverse teams and continue to improve internal processes and capabilities that are vital for enhancing nursing practice.

Future optimization efforts will include

- Streamlining documentation, on the basis of data and outcomes;
- Increasing clinical staff and manager proficiency to fully utilize the system's capabilities;
- Conducting research to achieve best practices; and
- Harnessing the power of electronic data capabilities to enable real-time reporting of information, interventions, and improvements in care.

Through our strong nursing leadership engagement and commitment, we have built a foundation of collaboration to continue our work. The challenge is to sustain it as we move through the next stage of our journey.

The key lessons we have taken away from our experience with implementing KP HealthConnect among nurses include

- Identify champions who are willing to dream big, abandon inefficient processes, and leave the "we've-always-done-it-that-way" comfort zone behind. They are critical leaders in selecting current and future features that have the functionality to enable improved nursing practices;
- Establish nursing governance early on, clarifying nursing strategy and vision; defining an overarching charter that includes roles, accountabilities, and expectations; and identifying decision-making processes;
- Involve nursing operations leadership with sustained commitment and engagement in the decision-making process wherever nursing practice, documentation, and workflow are affected;
- Involve front-line staff in the design as soon as possible, to ensure that content is meaningful to them. Otherwise, it will not be used. In the case of Kaiser Permanente, which has a large organized labor force, this meant working closely with our labor union partners to nurture and develop trust and positive working relationships;

- Start with a generalist approach in developing EHR clinical content, since the medical-surgical domain is the most prominent inpatient setting in terms of size and variability of patient demographics and conditions. This content can then be tailored to meet specialty needs while maintaining a core standard. Due to hospital workflows and patient care dynamics, inpatient content must be developed as an integrated system with appropriate touch points across physician documentation, orders, and nursing/interdisciplinary documentation;
- Maintain constant communication at all levels about the rationale behind content design or changes;
- Value the power of collaboration in building relationships and networked teams as the basis for achieving common goals. Challenging existing rules and having crucial conversations helps bridge across silos between disciplines, regions, facilities, or settings;
- Understand that technology alone will not transform nursing practice without work process redesign and a collaborative, learning culture;
- Know that the work of transformation and improvement never ends.

A CASE STUDY

DEPLOYING KP HEALTHCONNECT IN COLORADO

Enabling a Rapid and Successful Launch

By John H. Cochran, MD

The promise of information technology as an improvement tool in health care can only be realized long after the systems are selected, designed, and implemented. At that point, one comes to understand that success requires a greater focus on the commitment and enthusiasm of the people who will use the system than on the technology itself.

The importance of people and leadership in successfully deploying an electronic health record was one of the key learnings from the Colorado Permanente Medical Group's transition to KP HealthConnect in 2005. In that year, we faced the challenge of completing the entire implementation in one month—a seemingly impossible timeframe driven by the need to quickly replace an existing EHR system, which had been in place for seven years and was not functionally sustainable. Operating the old and new systems simultaneously was not a realistic option, so the speed of the transition was critical.

In Colorado, our journey with health IT had begun in the 1990s with an internally designed electronic health record system developed in partnership with a national vendor. A lot of time and energy had been spent in the development and design of this system before it was implemented over several months in 1998. Extensive user input had been part of the process of getting the product designed and built. Over

John H. Cochran, MD, served as medical director of the Colorado Permanente Medical Group during the implementation of KP HealthConnect. He is currently executive director of The Permanente Federation.

the next several years, the region learned to use the system and initiated the development of a disease registry to manage care in new and transformative ways.

In 2002, Kaiser Permanente's national leadership team, with the support of regional leaders, decided to adopt Epic System's electronic health record as the single national IT solution for all regions in both the ambulatory and inpatient settings. The Colorado region was scheduled to go live on KP HealthConnect in the fall of 2005. The rapid transition necessitated a strong commitment of physician leadership, focus, and support if we were to manage this disruptive and rapid change while maintaining access and performance in a very busy delivery system.

The requirement for speed in the context of a complex change environment meant that certain essential processes, competencies, and leadership behaviors had to be present from the outset. Balancing patient access and high standards of care against the need for a rapid system implementation is ultimately an artful process that draws on preparation and leadership. Following were the essential steps in the process.

Context Building

To ground a group of professionals in the need to make major, disruptive change, it is essential for leaders to share information and context about why this difficult change is essential. This is not a single convincing speech or memorandum. Rather, it is about a commitment to an iterative communication journey of proposing, listening, reacting, and learning in order to arrive at a shared understanding of why change is essential.

Building Capacity for Change

The design of the IT system should be optimized for the user. While there are limitations in "off-the-shelf" products such as the one purchased by Kaiser Permanente, the experience of the users is essential to inform modifications to the system. In our case, the development of the system involved a national "collaborative build" of the system's programs and clinical content (see Chapter Two). This involved regional users and national leadership teams working collaboratively to create a product that would meet the needs of each of the organization's eight regions, with a careful balance between national standardization and regional variation. This process, which continues to be used as we improve the system, optimizes the development of highly user-acceptable solutions.

There must also be commitment to provide extensive training in many formats. In addition to basic small-group class training, which was highly interactive and produced a strong sense of group learning, users were also offered DVDs and online training to help learn about the appearance and functionality of the system.

Throughout this process, we observed the development of a true learning community among our physicians and other clinicians as we progressed toward the go-live date.

Throughout the training, the commitment of leadership needs to be clear and visible, including support for physicians who bring both technical skills and clinical translational expertise to the training process. In addition, senior leaders must play a substantial role by demonstrating their own understanding and competence with the system. In our case, all senior leaders were expected to become accomplished users of the system and were visibly deployed to work in the clinics and departments as implementation proceeded. During the implementation, senior level leadership meetings were put on hold and leaders were strongly encouraged to stay out of their offices and be accessible in the clinics.

Clarity of Vision and Goal

Once the organization shares the context for change and adequately prepares users through training, senior leaders need to re-emphasize the vision and goals of the implementation clearly and without equivocation as the organization moves toward the initial launch. A clear and unwavering plan with milestones and deadlines helps to put everyone on notice about where to focus. We developed a very detailed implementation schedule that included additional "just-in-time" training.

To optimize opportunities to get off on the right foot, we carefully selected clinics for early deployment that we knew were staffed by eager "early adopters" who would most likely embrace the system, use it effectively, and be good models for other clinics to mirror. These early-adopter clinics provided a nucleus of super-users who became part of a human relay team that moved on to subsequent clinics in the deployment schedule to act as peer experts and share their knowledge of the nuances of the system with their colleagues. This ongoing process of having super-users visit each clinic was extremely valuable in demonstrating to new users how their peers were able to successfully use the system and rapidly return to seeing patients at a more normal pace.

Execution—Success—Trust—Momentum

After the first few clinics and departments began to use the system, a buzz of optimism began to develop among the various informal networks that were checking in to see if this was something that was going to crash and burn or go forward and result in a positive change. The region was communicating within itself an increasing level of confidence, enthusiasm, and trust, all of which were contributing to a growing sense of momentum. That momentum ultimately translated into an extraordinarily speedy deployment. But there is no question that the speed was made possible by all of the careful antecedent work—the context-setting, the clarity of goals, the training and capacity building, and the careful scheduling of early adopters and subsequent super-user support. All of it was essential to dispelling anxieties and skepticism and creating demand and enthusiasm among the clinicians to get the system up and running.

The KP HealthConnect deployment in Colorado took four weeks and two days—a remarkable achievement for a delivery system of more than eight hundred physicians working out of twenty-two medical offices and other facilities. Scott Smith, MD, one of the key leaders of the implementation, sent a voicemail to all clinicians as the implementation concluded, saying, "Thank you to all of you. You have just broken the world's record for deployment of an IT system. Welcome to the starting line."

Dr. Smith's point was that successful EHR deployment and user training is only the beginning of the real opportunity, which is to use the tool to transform the quality, service, and efficiency of health care delivery.

SECTION THREE

HARVESTING VALUE

CHAPTER FIVE

MAKING IT MATTER

Value and Quality

By Terhilda Garrido and Alide Chase

Chapter Summary

This chapter and the following chapters in Section Three address the issues of value realization in the implementation of an electronic health record (EHR)—the potential benefits in terms of quality of care, service, and system efficiency. Part One of this chapter, by Terhilda Garrido, discusses the basic conceptual framework for value realization in terms of immediate, short-term, and long-term benefits, and useful strategies for capturing them. Part Two of this chapter, by Alide Chase, focuses on how Kaiser Permanente prepared for maximizing the value of KP HealthConnect by reassessing and refocusing its entire quality infrastructure to ensure that its objectives and strategies aligned with the new capabilities available through the EHR.

Part One: Value Realization

After the long and sometimes arduous process of Kaiser Permanente HealthConnect implementation, Jack Cochran, MD, executive director of The Permanente Federation, congratulated the implementation teams for a job well done and then,

Terhilda Garrido, MPH, is vice president for strategic operations, National Quality & Care Delivery Excellence, at Kaiser Permanente. Alide Chase, MS, is Kaiser Permanente's senior vice president for quality and service.

borrowing a line from a colleague, quipped, "Welcome to the starting line." He was referring to the beginning of the process of value realization. Despite the enormous effort to implement an EHR, the accomplishment only achieved a necessary but insufficient condition for real change in health care. The process to achieve value—clinical quality improvement, operational efficiencies and cost savings, and improved consumer satisfaction—is neither straightforward nor easy. Certainly Kaiser Permanente has had its share of changes in direction and bumps along the way. However, the successes have indeed become evident and the potential is enormous.

The Challenges

The promise of EHR systems is enticing. They are viewed as key to improving the safety and quality of U.S. health care. A growing body of literature confirms their value in improving patient safety, coordination of care, and efficiency, as well as facilitating clinical decision making and adherence to evidence-based clinical guidelines (Kaushal, Shojania, and Bates, 2003). In addition, organizations have cited enhancements in billing and revenue collection (Thompson and others, 2007) and cost structure due to efficiencies in operational workflows.

However, for every story of success, there are examples of equivocal results, unexpected difficulties, or outright failure, about which we might observe: there are many ways to do a thing wrong.

It should be noted at the outset of this discussion that Kaiser Permanente's ability to maximize the benefits of KP HealthConnect have been shaped in important ways by the organization's highly integrated structure and its aligned financing system. The Congressional Budget Office has noted that "[i]n certain settings, health IT appears to make it easier to reduce health spending if other steps in the broader health care system are also taken to alter incentives to promote savings. By itself, the adoption of more health IT is generally not sufficient to produce significant cost savings" (Congressional Budget Office, 2008, p. 3).

The report goes on to note that integrated systems appear to be well suited to achieving benefits because of the alignment in goals and incentives across these organizations. For example, if Kaiser Permanente manages to reduce the level of clinical office visits because of the increased use of telephone visits and secure e-messages enabled by its information systems and patient demand, our physicians do not suffer financially, because all parts of the system—physicians, hospitals, and the health plan—have shared and aligned incentives to use a predetermined, capitated amount of members' premium dollars wisely. This is not necessarily the case in many health systems, in which medical groups, hospitals, and health plans operate independently of one another, often with conflicting incentives.

The natural advantage of integrated care organizations notwithstanding, other organizations in the less integrated, fee-for-service market can develop comprehensive incentives to allow for similar advantages. In the case of secure patient-physician e-messages, for instance, health plans could create an incentive for efficient, effective care by paying for coded, secure patient e-mails and improved patient outcomes.

Aligning Health IT and Quality Agendas

Kaiser Permanente employed a variety of techniques to encourage and set the stage for value realization. From its inception, the implementation of KP HealthConnect was aligned with Kaiser Permanente's quality and service improvement programs, including the development of Web-based health tools for members (see Chapter Eight). It was no coincidence that the health plan executive responsible for the implementation of KP HealthConnect was the same executive leading the organization's national efforts on the quality and service agenda. CEO George Halvorson hired Louise Liang, MD, to span both areas with the expectation that the health IT implementation would be well integrated with improvements in care and service.

Also, KP HealthConnect goals were established early in the project, with very strategic yet specific objectives designed to be consistent with Kaiser Permanente's aspirational commitment to providing care that would be high quality, personalized, convenient, and affordable. KP HealthConnect goals were designed to support these overarching commitments, as shown in Exhibit 5.1.

EXHIBIT 5.1. ALIGNING KP HEALTHCONNECT GOALS WITH KAISER PERMANENTE'S COMMITMENT TO MEMBERS.

High Quality of Care	Clinical information available 24/7 Unsurpassed clinical outcomes Real-time clinician access to recommended best practices National leadership in patient safety Enhanced research capabilities to support evidence-based care
Personal Care	Use of up-to-date clinical, social, and patient preference information Providing patients with information for shared decision making Enhanced personalized care
Convenient	Patient access to information via telephone, Web, and secure messaging Support for patients' participation in their own care Efficient access to care to minimize wait times and out-of-pocket costs Superior integration and continuity of care across specialists, settings, and time
Affordable	Reduced cost of care and improved visit experiences Elimination of waste associated with paper medical records Elimination of costly in-person services unless medically necessary or desired by the patient Streamlining IT and administrative processes and costs

The articulation of a Blue Sky Vision, as discussed in Chapter One, also helped to lift everyone's focus from a ground-level perspective on implementation issues to the larger and more exciting prospects of value and benefits.

A Framework for Value Realization

Wringing clear evidence of value out of new health IT tools is more challenging than one might suppose. In attempting to calculate the potential dollar value of Kaiser Permanente's investment in KP HealthConnect prior to implementation, the organization developed a full business case for the inpatient EHR and a partial business case for the outpatient EHR (Garrido and others, 2004). The process involved a national model that collected the best thinking (internal experience and external evidence weighed by operations experts) on benefits and allowed business and clinical units to interpret and select those benefits according to their sense of what they could deliver. In that admittedly theoretical exercise, we were able to show an 18 percent return on the investment. However, in dealing with real-world experience, the challenge has been in identifying savings that are directly attributable to KP HealthConnect. Given that the system is integrated with so many of our operational processes, many of which required workflow redesign, there are multiple factors involved in the value equation, and isolating the impact of KP HealthConnect is difficult, at best.

What is more, not all health IT value is created equal. We have found it useful to consider three categories of value, as displayed in Figure 5.1:

- Immediate, day-one value;
- Midterm value requiring harvesting; and
- Long-term transformation of care.

Approach to "Day One Value." The clinical use of KP HealthConnect provides immediate benefits to physicians and patients. The EHR, when fully integrated with a complete suite of ancillary systems, improves patient safety by ensuring that comprehensive, legible records are available immediately at every point of care within the system—at any time. It also eliminates duplicate lab and radiology tests by ensuring the availability of results. From a member service standpoint, having comprehensive information at every point of patient contact eliminates the annoyance of patients having to repeat the same information about allergies, medications, and other elements of their medical history every time they see a provider.

The key here is not to hinder the ability to achieve these benefits. For example, it is important to make sure that everyone providing care, including call centers and emergency departments, has access to the medical record. Also, the natural tendency of the informatics and IT staffs during implementation is to focus on provider usability and resuming operational workflows that have been disrupted. While these are important concerns, it is equally important to rethink and possibly redesign some of the standardized processes in lieu of restoring them. That, of course, is akin to changing the electrical system in a car that is being driven at 60 mph. In some cases, we automated less than

FIGURE 5.1. THREE PHASES OF VALUE REALIZATION.

III

Transformation of Care

II

Value Requiring Harvesting

I

Day One Value Created

The mere clinical use of KP HealthConnect gives us some benefits:

•Improved **patient safety** with **comprehensive, legible** records

•More efficient inpatient and outpatient care with 24/7 access to complete records

•Eliminates **duplicate lab/ radiology**/etc. tests by ensuring availability of results

•Improves providers' and Kaiser Permanente staff's ability to provide excellent **member service** by demonstrating "We know you"

Many benefits require deliberate policies, actions, and leadership:

•**Improved patient safety** due to implementation of level 1 drug-drug interaction alerts.

•**Reduced cost** of medical records operations

•Re-engineered **workflows** to improve quality outcomes while reducing waste and costs.

•Savings from legacy **system retirements**

•Reduced cost of **regulatory, compliance,** and other **reporting** activities

The full promise of KP HealthConnect comes with significantly more investment and leadership:

•Redefining a **new model of care** in which Web-enabled visits and home care replace many face-to-face visits

•Achieving the "**Blue Sky Vision**"

•An Information Hub (iHUB) **and common metrics** support identification and dissemination of operational **best practices and clinical guidelines** at an unprecedented rate

•Research and public health surveillance

optimal workflows and made a bad process worse. "Stabilization" of the system—or getting back to a baseline of performance—was required to fix some of the unintended consequences before we were able to move on fully to value realization.

Approach to "Value for Harvesting." Many benefits of KP HealthConnect have required deliberate policy changes, workflow redesign, focused and committed leadership, and/or an openness to entrepreneurial innovation on the part of knowledgeable clinicians. For example, improved patient safety can result from the implementation of Level 1 drug-drug interaction alerts. And chronic care management can be improved by electronic registries and EHRs that enable specialists to monitor and consult electronically in the primary care of entire populations of patients. But such benefits often require new workflows and possibly augmented and/or changed roles for care team members. As we like to say, "Expensive new technology plus old business processes equals expensive old business processes."

A good example of this type of benefit realization occurred in Kaiser Permanente's Hawaii region when nephrologist Brian J. Lee wanted to find a way to reach beyond the traditional individual patient referral process so that specialists could help monitor and manage the care offered to an entire population of 10,000 patients with chronic kidney disease. He and his colleagues designed a quality improvement pilot, using an electronic database of lab results to identify and rank for risk all chronic kidney disease patients.

Using KP HealthConnect, Lee electronically monitors the primary care delivered to the most high-risk patients to ensure it is in line with evidence-based treatment recommendations and, whenever appropriate, provides unsolicited e-consults to the patients' primary care physicians. In effect, he turned the referral system on its head. In many cases, Lee recommended that patients be referred to a nephrologist for more intensive care. In others, the primary care physician was given the treatment recommendations necessary to prevent the need for referral. Making this inverted referral system work required not only the patients' electronic records, but dramatic changes in the relationship between specialists and primary care physicians, as well as the active support of clinical leadership.

Results of Lee's five-year project showed that it increased early intervention for high-risk patients and reduced by two-thirds the number of late specialist referrals—those occurring within four months of the onset of end-stage renal disease. Such early referral is essential, Lee explained, in order to make changes that will slow the progress of the disease.

"Management of patients with chronic kidney disease or other conditions requires comprehensive information technology," said Lee. "The advent of KP HealthConnect in Hawaii in 2005 meant that more data were available in electronic form (blood pressure, weight, updated drug lists) to be pulled into our database and that any patient's entire medical record was available immediately if we needed more information than our database provided" (Lee and Forbes, 2009).

Approach to Transforming Care.

Kaiser Permanente is still learning what is possible with KP HealthConnect and its Web-based member portal, called My Health Manager. We are on a very long journey. We have not yet fully realized the right approach to transformation, but we believe the components must include the following:

- *Aligned incentives*—There should be clarity that what improves the overall health care system ultimately benefits all components of the system (doctors, hospitals, health plans, and, most important, the patient and member).
- *A shared vision*—Four years after the creation of the Blue Sky Vision, Kaiser Permanente executives were interviewed to understand if the premise set forth was still relevant, and the consensus was a resounding yes: patient empowerment, quality of care, member service, leveraging our technology to allow for efficient and effective processes of care—all had become part of the organizational DNA.
- *Capability to identify, support, and disseminate care innovations*—Encouraging innovation and learning at all levels of the organization and having a format for sharing these innovations supports the ability to engage providers and staff in care transformation. Later in this and the following chapters of this section, we relate other examples of this type of innovation and how they have been shared across the organization.
- *Collaboration and cultural transformation*—A consistent application of new health IT tools has helped Kaiser Permanente's far-flung regions and providers overcome some of the limits of isolation and resistance to innovations "not invented here." A good example of how our clinical culture changed, related in Chapter Six, is the story of our Inter-regional Oncology Chiefs Group, representing hundreds of oncologists, which came to an historic agreement to work across regions to define and share a common set of clinical, evidence-based protocols that would be embedded into one single build for the KP HealthConnect Oncology module (called Beacon®).
- *Leadership support*—Successful care transformation requires new levels of cooperation among regional and national clinical operations leaders and essential support for local and regional innovations. The success stories related throughout this book would not have been possible without the visible and sustained support of these operations leaders.
- *Not standing in front of fast-moving trains*—We have witnessed a genuine sea-change in ambulatory care as patient interactions via telephone or secure e-messaging have come to account for 41 percent—and growing—of primary care patient contacts. The availability of the secure patient-physician messaging functionality presented our physicians with many questions and concerns, but the medical group leadership embraced the notion that, in the end, it would contribute to more convenient and better care for the patient.

- *Free the data*—Critical to ultimate transformation is and will be the use of the mountain of data that KP HealthConnect collects and stores. We are still very much in the process of harnessing and mining that data. Every day we have more examples of the potential improvements it makes possible—cutting-edge research, new clinical outcome reporting, new operations reporting, new information to better understand patients' health needs and preferences, and improved monitoring for patient safety risks.

Essential EHR Functions Supporting Value Realization

- Automated and organized information at the point of clinical care—all patients, all contacts, all the time
- Supporting clinical decision making:
  - Alerts
  - Templates for documentation as well as evidence-based guidelines for care
  - Functionality supporting consistency in reliable care workflows
- Expanding and streamlining modalities of care for patient convenience and empowerment:
  - Effective telephone visits
  - Secure e-messages
  - Web services and access to personal health record information
  - Patient information entered into the EHR by patients
- Population care tools for inreach and outreach
- Use of data coming from EHRs for
  - New clinical evidence base
  - New health services/operations insights
  - Rapid, robust clinical research
- Use of data for predictive modeling

Leveraging Value Through Information Sharing and Knowledge Management

With the implementation of KP HealthConnect, Kaiser Permanente's culture underwent significant change from siloed regional and clinical practices to an organization with national purpose and vision, and national health IT tools to enable them. Improvements in local medical care practices and workflow could now be shared more readily, and a common language and lexicon developed. This commonality, while imperfect and incomplete, has allowed for the sharing of successful practices that add value across the program, taking Kaiser Permanente a big step forward as a "learning organization." Several mechanisms were important in promoting this change.

SmartBook for Value Realization/Optimization. To support local and regional operations' work in achieving strategic plan targets for quality, member service, and efficiency, we created the KP HealthConnect SmartBook for Value Realization and Optimization, which is maintained by a small national department that provides evaluation and analysis of potential health IT benefits. The SmartBook (see sample page in Figure 5.2) is an online, searchable compendium of information on demonstrated best practices for quality, cost management, revenue enhancement, and other potential benefits to be realized through the full implementation of KP HealthConnect in concert with other actions.

Each SmartBook "page" outlines a specific area of opportunity. Currently we have published more than 250 opportunities, each of which identifies levers for harvesting value from KP HealthConnect, such as changes in workflow, potential impacts that may be expected from using the lever, resources to contact for further information and support, and the basis or evidence for the impact estimates. As we learn from each region's experience in utilizing different components of KP HealthConnect, we

FIGURE 5.2. SAMPLE SMARTBOOK PAGE.

New for v6.0

Opportunity: Pharmacy

Confidence Level

Lever: Implement the Tamoxifen/antidepressant Best Practice Alert (BPA) to prevent drug interactions that increase breast cancer reoccurrence.

"Evidence"/Expert Opinion/Basis: NCAL and the NW region have implemented the interregional collaborative Tamoxifen/antidepressant BPA to address medication safety issues identified by the Institute of Medicine and the Institute for Safe Medication Practices.

The **Interregional Decision Support Subcommittee (DSSC)** developed the Tamoxifen/antidepressant BPA in KP HealthConnect in 2009 as part of ongoing work with new drug interaction and drug condition alerts.

This alert notifies clinicians that they need to avoid the use of antidepressants in women who are prescribed Tamoxifen.

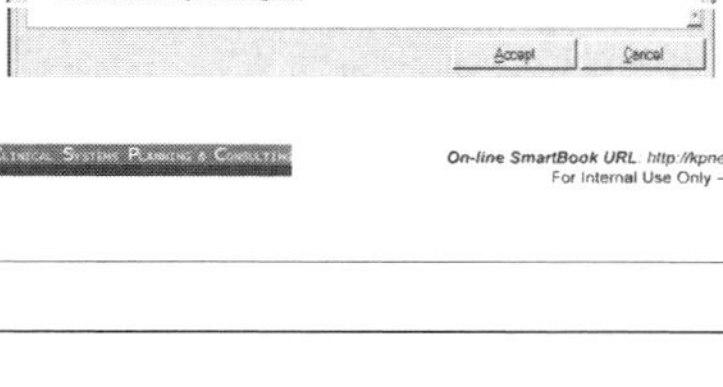

Source	• Drug FAQs for Clinicians – Frequently asked Questions, 2009. Michael Krall, MD
Key Assumptions	Benefit level assumptions: • Alert infrastructure is in place within region • Medication safety groups are engaged in KPHC activities Benefit realization time: 2 weeks
Key Enablers	• Strong leadership with decision making authority and ability to operationalize changes in practice • Strong safety and quality culture • Metrics and feedback mechanisms to enable quality improvement and performance management
KPHC Functionality	• KPHC Clinicals – Ambulatory and Inpatient (electronic prescribing)
Contact	• Michael Krall, MD – NW Physician Lead for Clinical Content and Decision Support, Interregional Decision Support Lead • David Campen, MD - Medical Director-Drug Information Utilization and Technology

"There is an increased focus on medication safety at the national level. KP needs to leverage all systems so that the right person gets the right medication at the right time in a way that is safe for that patient. The benefit of KP HealthConnect is that patients have one common medical profile so we can make sure the oncologist treating a breast cancer patient and the psychiatrist treating depression are given information to maximize the effectiveness of the medications to prevent a potential reoccurrence of breast cancer.

This alert leverages KP HealthConnect to bring critical information to prescribers at a time when they need it most."

David Campen, MD Medical Director-Drug Information Utilization and Technology

Clinical Systems Planning & Consulting

On-line SmartBook URL: *http://kpnet.kp.org/kphealthconnect/stabilize/smartbook/index.htm*
For Internal Use Only – Proprietary & Confidential – Version 6.0

#00373

continually update the SmartBook with new levers updating benefit estimates as well as successful practices. The pages are available to clinicians and operations management on our Kaiser Permanente intranet site and in hardcopy.

Inter-Regional Webinars and Shared Learning Sessions. There is no substitute for live information sharing and networking to create momentum. Kaiser Permanente sponsors a variety of internal webinars, virtual user conferences, and regular organization-wide conferences to allow interested parties to learn from innovative operational leaders showcasing their work and results.

Internal and External Journal Evaluations. The power of rigorous quantitative evaluations focused on critical areas of KP HealthConnect impact has been very important to Kaiser Permanente's progress in value realization. The sharing of these evaluations internally has been valuable in building support and credibility among clinicians and others for the sometimes difficult adjustments required for value realization, and sharing them with external audiences is essential to the organization's non-profit commitment to community knowledge. A particularly effective way to reach both the internal and external audiences has been publication of our evaluation research in our own quarterly medical journal, *The Permanente Journal,* and in various other national, peer-reviewed medical and health policy journals. Sometimes, reading an evaluation of a system in an independent, third-party journal carries greater credibility among internal stakeholders than the same information presented in an internal conference or webinar. For a select listing of published, peer-reviewed evaluations of KP HealthConnect, see the Appendix.

Monitoring and Tracking Impact. Sharing with clinicians the impact of KP Health-Connect on all aspects of health care delivery is vital for driving change and value realization. One of our most important tools for this is the periodic "Core Value Metrics" report, produced by an internal group of data analysts who focus on mining and interpreting EHR and other related systems data for learnings about care delivery. The power of this tracking is shown in Figure 5.3, on usage of KP HealthConnect's "After Visit Summary" (AVS). The AVS is a paper summary of the patient's information (allergies, current medications, physician instructions, and so on) that is given to the patient at the end of his or her visit. Polling data indicates there is significant improvement in patient satisfaction when the AVS is distributed and reviewed with patients by their doctors—a finding that was published in the KP Smart-Book. It has also been associated with improved patient compliance with treatment plans. Initially, the use of AVS by doctors was inconsistent and generally low level. By tracking AVS usage along with dissemination of the evidence of impact on patient satisfaction and compliance in the SmartBook, AVS usage has increased considerably.

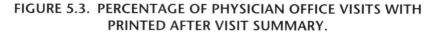

FIGURE 5.3. PERCENTAGE OF PHYSICIAN OFFICE VISITS WITH
PRINTED AFTER VISIT SUMMARY.

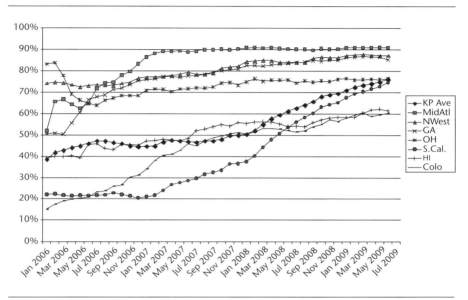

Part Two: Reassessing the Quality Agenda with KP HealthConnect

Many of the advances achieved with KP HealthConnect have been dependent not only on the technology but, just as important, on a closely related realignment of Kaiser Permanente's quality and service focus, including the Blue Sky Vision commitment to patient-centeredness. Indeed, without a concerted effort to match our quality goals, infrastructure, accountabilities, and culture to the potential inherent in the new technology, KP HealthConnect would fall far short of our overriding goal to transform care. Reviewing, revising, and renewing our approach to quality was essential in laying the foundation upon which KP HealthConnect could enable a transformation of care delivery.

During 2003 through 2004, the organization's senior executives took on the challenge of strengthening the national quality agenda and related infrastructure. CEO George Halvorson led this work by appointing to the board of directors very strong, involved individuals with a keen appetite for performance oversight in the areas of quality, service, and patient safety. The fact that far more needed to be done was evident at the conclusion of a board meeting when, having spent hours reviewing a four-inch binder of metrics on quality performance, one knowledgeable member asked, "So, how are we doing?" Clearly, we needed a paradigm shift in how to prioritize, measure, and communicate our quality and service performance.

Reassessing Quality Systems for EHR Alignment

The board's quality committee, under the leadership of Christine Cassel, MD, president and CEO of the American Board of Internal Medicine and the ABIM Foundation, began a multiyear improvement approach that was initiated by a total system quality assessment. The objectives included determinations of quality structures and processes in place; assessment of their robustness, effectiveness, and linkages; identification of gaps or redundancies in the processes and the information produced; and determination of steps needed to ensure that Kaiser Permanente could meet its commitment to quality.

Louise Liang, MD, the senior executive for quality in the health plan, dubbed the Quality Systems Assessment the "Sarbanes-Oxley for quality." The work involved navigating through uncharted waters for a multihospital integrated delivery system of the size and complexity of Kaiser Permanente. But in 2003, with the support of ECRI, a research organization nationally known for technology assessment, health policy, and research, and our own audit and compliance organizations, an organization-wide quality assessment was conducted.

Among the assessment's key recommendations were that we strengthen and clarify the system-wide performance expectations and goals, cascade them through the entire organization, build a robust national quality infrastructure, and create clear lines of accountability at local, regional, and national levels. In an organization where regional autonomy had long been held as one of the highest organizational values, this was a new way of thinking. The accountability shift from "We believe we deliver the highest quality care" to "the numbers tell the real story" was a long time coming and one that is still evolving today.

However, the stage was set for such a change when the organization's national and regional quality leaders, representing the medical groups as well as the health plan and hospitals, joined to replace the existing national quality oversight structures with a new National Quality Committee. This enabled leaders from across the organization to examine both regional and system-wide quality performance data together, thus developing deepening respect for each other's challenges and sharpening the passion for system-wide improvement. The heightened emphasis on quality improvement also sparked the establishment of three-year, system-wide goals, including a commitment to reach the 90th percentile on all HEDIS and hospital (Joint Commission) quality measures. Accountability for performance was reinforced by tying the goals to executive and management compensation incentive structures and the pay-for-performance programs with the organization's labor union partners.

Safe Implementation Before Quality Improvement

Even though it was clear that the Blue Sky Vision called for a high-quality, patient-centered health care system, the initial emphasis in KP HealthConnect deployment focused on achieving operational efficiencies, creating an effective communication system among clinicians, and learning to use the tool itself. Operations leaders were charged with the challenging task of "keeping the lights on" during the deployment. The execution plan for KP HealthConnect implementation required the full attention of operations leaders. Comments such as "We cannot be distracted with new or additional work right now; all we can do is focus on a safe implementation," were heard frequently across the organization.

As a consequence, the push for new levels of improvement in quality performance had to take a back seat to the demands of the initial deployment of KP HealthConnect. The thinking was that improvement could come more quickly after providers and staff gained confidence in using the system. Some clinical processes and workflows were redesigned prior to implementation, particularly in the inpatient setting, and some during implementation, but many had to wait until full implementation was completed. In hindsight, we believe there was wisdom in our hybrid approach, in that providers were able to identify new and different ways of using the tool as they became increasingly confident in its use.

As organizational confidence in the use of KP HealthConnect grew, expectations about achieving leading performance in the areas of clinical outcomes, safety, and service returned to the forefront, especially for operations leaders, who increasingly assumed ownership of the quality agenda. Early thinking about the ways the EHR could support quality improvement matured into the development of sophisticated panel management support tools (see Chapter Six) to move to reality the national goal of leading in preventive services, management of chronic conditions, and early cancer detection.

On Training Quality Leaders in IT

One of our many small "ah-ha" moments along the quality and EHR journey was the realization that we, as quality leaders, needed to become IT-sophisticated business leaders. In the past, it was acceptable for quality to have very little knowledge of the building components and capabilities of our IT systems. We left that to the IT group and to our clinical informatics physicians and nurses whom we expected to translate our magical thinking into reality. Since so much of the daily clinical operations is driven by KP HealthConnect, and we rely on workflows to ensure highly reliable care, we know now that quality leaders need an intimate knowledge of the system's capabilities. Our current challenge is finding a training approach that effectively meets that need—most existing training programs focus on the daily user of the system. The "IT sophisticated" quality leader will have enough knowledge to ask good, probing questions of the IT staff on capabilities, have a reasonably accurate sense of data that should be reportable from the system, and have an understanding of the EHR tools available to clinicians and patients.

— Ruth Brentari, senior director, Department of Care & Service Quality

New Approaches to Viewing and Understanding Quality Data

Meanwhile, in 2005, with the growing national demand for transparency on health care quality, the organization created a national "dashboard" that reported quality, service, safety, risk management, and resource stewardship in the hospitals and ambulatory clinics (see Figure 5.4). Prior to this effort, system-wide reporting had consisted of hundreds of measures being presented at different times during the year. The new dashboard, developed with the Institute for Healthcare Improvement and known internally as "Big Q," integrated several concepts: whole-system measures; full transparency of performance; comparison to external benchmarks; and integration of clinical quality, delivery system satisfaction, patient safety, and affordability into one shared view. Even during development, it was recognized that additional measures would be added as the ability to extract more outcomes data directly from KP HealthConnect became available.

The increased transparency in reporting served as a powerful catalyst for change. The ability for leaders to see their performance benchmarked against the best in class externally and internally tapped a natural sense of competition and the will to improve. Hospital executives were able to quickly identify top performers and seek guidance on what factors lead to their success. Lower performers could also be easily identified, and customized approaches were developed to support their improvement. Conversations among operations leaders and even board members quickly moved from anecdotal evidence of quality to deeper, data-driven reviews and expectations for action and improvement.

The new depth and comparative presentation of data, much of it enabled by KP HealthConnect, meant that the executive vice president for health plan and hospital operations, Bernard Tyson, could incorporate a complete profile of each hospital on his site visits throughout the organization. He reported that he was able to celebrate successes and ask questions about key areas of performance on the basis of much richer information. After four years of use, the performance in every whole-system measure has significantly improved—specifically, a significant drop in hospital mortality and patient harm, an improvement in HEDIS and cost of care rates, and an improvement in hospital and outpatient service performance. In some cases, the speed of improvement has outperformed the organizational goal for that year.

While the Big Q has served its purpose to help the board and managers track the progress in system-wide performance, we augmented the composites, rates, and indexes with more human-scale information to drive commitment to the work. Following the advice of the Institute for Healthcare Improvement, multiyear goals were translated from

FIGURE 5.4. THE "BIG Q" QUALITY DASHBOARD (NOVEMBER 2009).

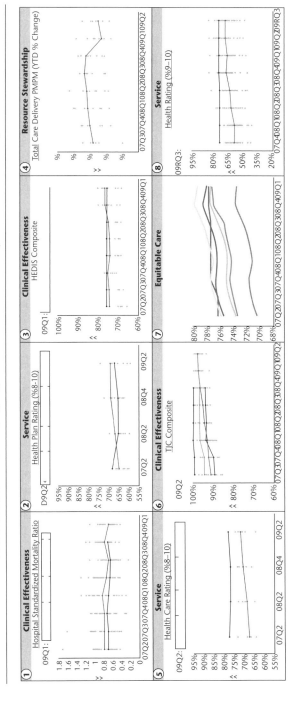

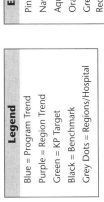

The "Big Q" Quality Dashboard integrates a broad range of whole-system measures on clinical quality, delivery system satisfaction, patient safety, and affordability into a single view. The graphs illustrate progress in clinical effectiveness, safety, resource stewardship, equitable care, and service.

rates and improvement in index scores to numbers of lives saved and harm prevented (see Exhibit 5.2). The shift in language served to align front-line, middle, and senior leaders in the three-year march toward transformational improvement in the care delivery system.

The next step in transparency and data integration was to move beyond the traditional clinical quality perspective and add information on cost savings or resource stewardship. Defining quality results in terms of both dollar savings and lives saved was a new way of thinking about the shared accountability for overall performance (see Exhibit 5.3). It also reflected a conviction that high quality is frequently less costly.

EXHIBIT 5.2. TRANSLATING CLINICAL METRICS TO LIVES SAVED, 2004–2008 Q4.

Metric	Increase	Savings per Decade
Cholesterol Control	16.8%	1,350 Lives
Blood Pressure Control	36.6 %	4,890 Lives
HbA1C <9.0	7.8%	738 Lives
Smoking Cessation	14.0%	787 Lives
Breast Cancer Screening	11.3%	565 Lives
		4,349 Stage 4 Cases Prevented
Cervical Cancer Screening	5.8%	38 Lives
Colon Cancer Screening	24.2%	3,838 Lives
Total		12,206 Lives Saved

EXHIBIT 5.3. LINKING QUALITY IMPROVEMENTS WITH FINANCIAL OUTCOMES.

Potential Savings from Reducing Harm	
Estimated savings by reducing LOS cost for MRSA, C Diff, and urinary tract infections	$34,000,000
Estimated savings based on extrapolated CMS costs for coded harm from falls and coded pressure ulcers	$17,000,000
Potential savings from medication reconciliation on admission	$9,000,000
Annualized savings estimate of reducing costs associated with BSI, VAP, and surgical site infections	$8,000,000
Conservative savings estimate (10 percent of admission savings) Above from med reconciliation at transfer, discharge, and other indirect savings	$900,000
Total (projected savings may be incremental, as some processes are already in place and achieving impact)	$68,900,000

In 2008, the organization's strategic plan placed the transformation of the care delivery system as the top priority. The shift in attention to this aspirational goal of total delivery system transformation cannot be overstated, and without the simultaneous implementation of KP HealthConnect and the renewal of the quality agenda, it would not have been imaginable. The stage had been set, the expectations were clear, and the shift of ownership for quality performance from quality department leaders to operations and senior leaders was in full swing.

The People Behind the Quality Dashboard

Electronic health records—and their associated data extraction frameworks—require a governance infrastructure in order to fully realize the benefits of electronic data for quality improvement, research, and general health care analytics. Early in the development of Big Q, we recognized the need for a steering committee to address policy and strategic direction.

The steering committee addresses fundamental governance questions, including the granting of access privileges to users outside Kaiser Permanente, the recommendation of numeric targets for specific performance measures, and decisions on sponsoring and/or funding specialized views for stakeholder groups such as nursing, infection control, and palliative care.

A technical workgroup comprising measurement, analytical, and programming experts in the quality and IT departments provides guidance to the steering committee on informatics or complex methodological questions. The technical workgroup also recommends methodologies for aggregating individual metrics into broader composites, identifies options for weighting individual components of the composites, provides solutions for depicting measurement uncertainty or imprecision in graphical displays, optimizes navigation within the dashboard (minimizing keystrokes required to "roll up" or "drill down"), and promotes consistency in visual displays across the dashboard's different domains.

Both the steering committee and the technical workgroup have clinical members or advisors to provide guidance on the strength and quality of the evidence underlying the performance measures in the dashboard, helping to ensure that the dashboard remains a credible source of performance across key dimensions of quality.

— Andy Amster, director, Center for Healthcare Analytics, Kaiser Permanente

The following quality performance charts (Figures 5.5 and 5.6) offer what we believe is compelling evidence that we are now well on our way to achieving the goal of system transformation.

FIGURE 5.5. SCREENING RATES FOR BREAST, COLORECTAL, AND CERVICAL CANCER.

Cancer Screening

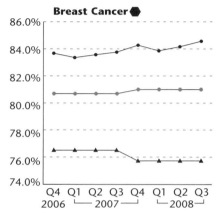

Exceed the national 90th percentile
for Breast Cancer Screening.

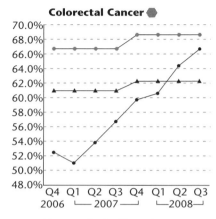

Have made significant improvements
in Colorectal Cancer Screening and
we now approach the national 90th
percentile.

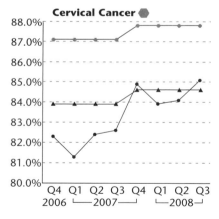

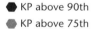

Have made improvements in Cervical
Cancer Screening, moving above the
national 75th percentile.

FIGURE 5.6. PERFORMANCE IN THREE CHRONIC CARE MEASURES: BLOOD PRESSURE, CARDIOVASCULAR LDL CONTROL, AND DIABETES LDL CONTROL.

Chronic Care

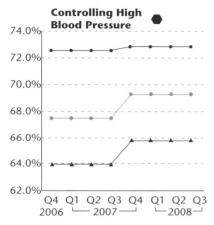

Exceed the national 90th percentile in Controlling High Blood Pressure.

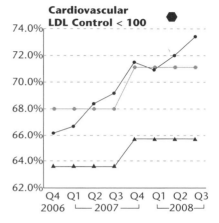

Have made significant improvements in the Cardiovascular LDL Control < 100 measure with performance now exceeding the national 90th percentile.

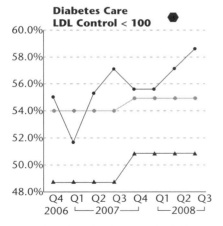

Continued to improve the Diabetes Care LDL Control < 100 measure with performance now exceeding the national 90th percentile.

CHAPTER SIX

MANAGING THE HEALTH OF POPULATIONS

By Louise L. Liang, MD; Robert Unitan, MD; and Jed Weissberg, MD

Chapter Summary

This chapter discusses ways in which KP HealthConnect is being used to enable significantly improved population care management—the key strategy for addressing the most debilitating and costly chronic conditions. Part One of this chapter, by Louise Liang, MD, describes the conceptual basis of population care management and how the advent of the electronic health record (EHR) is enabling the unleashing of its full promise. It concludes with several case studies of chronic condition care innovations enabled by KP HealthConnect. Part Two of this chapter, by Robert Unitan, MD, describes a unique application of the EHR's population management functionality that allows primary care physicians, without any analytic assistance, to proactively manage the health needs of their entire practice of patients, focusing both on individuals and on condition-specific cross-sections of their patient populations. In Part Three, Jed Weissberg, MD, discusses how various clinical specialty groups at Kaiser Permanente have seized on new IT functionalities to promote closer clinical collaboration among physicians in separate regions and developed new EHR-based applications for quality improvement in their specialty areas.

Louise L. Liang, MD, is the retired senior vice president for Quality and Clinical Systems Support in Kaiser Permanente's national office; Robert Unitan, MD, is director of operations, Medical Specialties, Kaiser Permanente-Northwest; and Jed Weissberg, MD, is the current senior vice president for Quality and Care Delivery Excellence in Kaiser Permanente's national office and former associate executive director for Quality of The Permanente Federation of medical groups.

Part One: Fulfilling the Promise of Population Care Management

Health information technology in general and Kaiser Permanente HealthConnect in particular are enabling Kaiser Permanente to deliver as never before on the long-held but largely unfulfilled promise of population care management—the systematic care of entire subpopulations of patients who share common medical conditions.

Prior to the implementation of electronic health records, the concept and practice of population care management was more an aspiration than a reality. Within any large patient population there are subsets of individuals who share certain conditions or diseases—many of them high-cost and high-prevalence chronic conditions such as cardiovascular disease, diabetes, asthma, depression, and cancer. The goal in identifying and caring for these subpopulations is to systematically target them with evidence-based care interventions that improve or maintain their health status and reduce the chances that they will progress to more debilitating and expensive stages of illness. Many health care organizations have relied on patient registries to track patients with these specific diagnoses, usually with data gleaned from various IT or administrative systems such as lab, pharmacy, or insurance claims.

The ability to more efficiently and completely identify these populations and develop effective common care protocols holds great opportunity for improving the nation's overall health outcomes and containing rapidly rising costs. Nearly half of all Americans have at least one chronic condition, and half of this group has multiple chronic conditions (Thorpe, 2006). Treatment of patients with chronic conditions accounts for close to 80 percent of the nation's total health care costs (Robert Wood Johnson Foundation & Partnership for Solutions, 2004). Many of these conditions are fully preventable, and all of them are progressive, yet their progress can be slowed or arrested by appropriate, timely treatment.

Lack of Systems Holds Back the Promise

Unfortunately, the record for effective treatment of these diseases has been disappointing. The well-known Rand study on how well recommended care processes are followed for thirty acute and chronic conditions documented that only 56.1 percent of chronic disease patients receive recommended care (McGlynn and others, 2003). This is partly because identifying and tracking these patients without an EHR is labor intensive and unreliable, and partly because the recommended care guidelines are not accessible to most physicians at the point of care. Also, the necessary coordination among the various providers who participate in the care of chronic disease patients is absent or insufficiently timely, as is the continuous follow-up and feedback between patients and providers required for effective disease management. These critical gaps permit important warning signs to go unnoticed and therefore untreated, often resulting in unnecessary complications and acute care crises.

Effective care management requires *systems* of care that remain unavailable to the large majority of health care providers. Such systems go far beyond the capabilities or resources of any individual physician. The processes involve the systematic coordination of multidisciplinary care teams, including primary care and specialty physicians, nurses, nutritionists, social workers, and others. They also require the ability to develop and implement condition-specific, evidence-based care guidelines, or pathways, and to regularly monitor and measure the health status of both the entire subgroup and its individual members. And finally, these systems ultimately depend for success on the routine education of patients and on the engagement of patients in their own care, most of which takes place outside the usual one-on-one patient-physician office visit.

In the earliest days of care management, chronic care protocols and other best practice information were printed in fat binders and summarized on printed pocket cards and distributed to physicians. Their impact, not surprisingly, was minimal, as physicians had neither the time nor the ability to look up complex care guidelines when they most needed them—in their one-on-one encounters with individual patients. What's more, the highly coordinated team care was nearly impossible to achieve without a means of sharing and accessing up-to-date, accurate patient information whenever and wherever it was needed.

The development of early versions of EHRs in most of Kaiser Permanente's regions in the 1990s represented an important coming of age for the care management approach. Clinical IT systems of various levels of sophistication and functionality were developed to automatically identify members of chronic disease subgroups and to stratify those populations according to the severity of their conditions and health care needs. Individuals at the highest risk levels could be identified for intensive care management approaches overseen by dedicated care management staff, while those at lower levels of severity or risk could receive more health education and preventive care, including self-care. These systems included condition-specific, evidence-based care guidelines and decision-support tools for point-of-service prompts and alerts to physicians. In Kaiser Permanente, they were developed by clinicians at the regional level in collaboration with the organization's Care Management Institute (CMI), created in 1997 as the central gathering point for studying and creating evidence-based care protocols.

Experience with these regional IT systems provided convincing evidence that EHRs could be effective in helping physicians reduce unnecessary variations in care and improve quality. For instance, an internal report showed that before the evidence-based guideline on upper gastrointestinal radiology tests was embedded in the physician ordering system of KP HealthConnect's predecessor EHR in the Northwest region, only 55 percent of all orders for such tests conformed to the recommendations in the evidence-based care guideline. After the guideline was embedded in the EHR, 86 percent to 90 percent of all tests conformed to the guideline. In addition, the number of such tests ordered declined by 40 percent—a strong indication that the guideline was helping clinicians make better judgments about when a relatively invasive medical procedure was really needed and when it was not.

However, while each region developed its own approaches to care management based on the unique scope and functionality of its information systems, from an organization-wide perspective it remained a patchwork of practices, with continuing wide variations in care and health outcomes among the regions.

The EHR—Enabling the Full Promise of Care Management

The implementation of a single, integrated EHR, KP HealthConnect, across all Kaiser Permanente regions starting in 2004 has represented a true milestone in care management at Kaiser Permanente—the ability to transform that variable patchwork of systems into a finely woven fabric of common, evidence-based approaches and tools for chronic conditions that covers 8.6 million members with a degree of consistency, effectiveness, and efficiency not realized before.

While it is still too early to draw detailed analysis of the value of KP HealthConnect across the spectrum of chronic care management, it is clear that it has been a powerful contributor in pushing Kaiser Permanente to the top rankings for HEDIS, the national standard for health care performance developed by the National Committee for Quality Assurance.

According to the 2008 HEDIS performance data (the most recently available as this book was going to press), one or more Kaiser Permanente regions topped the nation in eight overall measures. In the management of diabetic nephropathy, for example, our Hawaii region was number one in the country. The Northern California and Colorado regions were tied for third place, and six of the eight Kaiser Permanente regions were ranked among the top eight nationwide. Every Kaiser Permanente region was the HEDIS leader for nephropathy in its area of the country. Organization-wide, Kaiser Permanente ranked in the 90th percentile among all health plans in our internally generated HEDIS composite of thirty-three clinical care measures.

What's more, the process of clinicians from all the Kaiser Permanente regions joining together with CMI to design and build the clinical content to support key care management capabilities into KP HealthConnect produced an invaluable byproduct. For the first time in anyone's memory, operations and clinical leaders developed a system-wide vision of what care management can look like and accomplish in an integrated delivery system serving 8.6 million members. And that common vision continues to serve as a foundation for unprecedented levels of collaboration and shared learning.

Case Studies in EHR-Enabled Care Management

Following are three case studies illustrating how use of KP HealthConnect and related health IT tools have enabled innovative quality improvements in the prevention and treatment of chronic diseases and other important health needs.

Getting to the Heart of the Problem: Coronary Artery Disease (CAD). Coronary artery disease is one of the top five chronic conditions that account for the majority of health care costs. It is the leading cause of death in the United States, affecting sixty-one million Americans and contributing to 40 percent of all deaths. Studies show that secondary prevention strategies can dramatically reduce CAD morbidity and mortality, but there still remains a large "treatment gap" between recommended, evidence-based care and the actual care received by most CAD patients.

Kaiser Permanente-Colorado's Collaborative Cardiac Care Service (CCCS) has been able to prevent chronic conditions such as CAD from becoming life-threatening crises. The initiative enlists virtually every hospitalized CAD patient in both short- and long-term care management programs, conducted by teams of registered nurses and clinical pharmacists.

Within twenty-four hours of hospital discharge, all patients who have been hospitalized for a cardiac event are enrolled in a three- to six-month educational and case management cardiac rehabilitation program focused on behavioral changes and secondary prevention strategies. This phase of the program is conducted by nurses via regularly scheduled phone calls, in-person group visits, and routine clinic visits, and emphasizes behavioral strategies and adherence to cholesterol-lowering medications. Detailed, individualized care plans are prepared in KP HealthConnect and discussed with every patient and regularly reviewed and updated at every patient contact.

In the follow-up phase, all patients are assigned a clinical pharmacy specialist who manages the patient's medication regimen. The pharmacists ensure that patients are evaluated and started on beta-blockers and daily aspirin, and order laboratory tests to monitor the efficacy and safety of medications. They also provide ongoing behavior change support, if required. All patient information is shared among all care givers through KP HealthConnect.

KP HealthConnect serves as the hub of all CCCS patient information. A related Web-based database—the "population tool," used for scheduling appointments and lab tests—allows team members to track all patients, identify those who have missed scheduled tests, and remind them to reschedule. These health IT tools enable CCCS teams to access patient information, ensure adherence to care protocols, coordinate care with primary care physicians and cardiologists, and follow individualized treatment plans.

Between 1996 and 2004, CAD patients who were enrolled in the program for an average 3.5 years experienced a 76 percent reduction in death from any cause and a 73

percent reduction from cardiac-related deaths, compared to patients who did not participate in the program. Increases in survival rates were even greater for patients who enrolled
soon after a cardiac event and stayed in the program continuously. In practical terms, it is
estimated that more than 280 costly emergency interventions were prevented each year.
Due in large measure to the cardiac care program, in 2007 Kaiser Permanente-Colorado's
HEDIS scores placed the region in the 90th percentile in the nation for cholesterol control,
number two in the nation for cholesterol screening in CAD patients, and number four in
the nation for continued use of beta-blockers in post-heart-attack patients. The program
also was awarded the Care Continuum Alliance's Leadership Award in 2009 for the best
use of technology toward achieving and maintaining improved health outcomes.

Mammography Screening: Operation Innovation. On the basis of rates from
2004–2006, 12.7 percent of women born today will be diagnosed with cancer of the
breast at some time during their lifetime (Ries and others, 2006). However, early mammography screening, detection, diagnosis, and treatment can reduce the death rate by
20 to 50 percent, since more than 96 percent of all early stage, localized breast cancers
are curable. That said, studies show that due to fear, lack of information, lack of access,
and other reasons, many women are not screened at the recommended age or intervals,
or are not receiving timely diagnosis following positive screening results.

Recognizing the seriousness of these issues, Kaiser Permanente launched a campaign to identify and contact—by any and all means—all women who meet the age
recommendation for mammograms and have not been screened within the past eighteen months. The campaign, called Operation Innovation, was first launched and
tested in Kaiser Permanente's Southern California region and subsequently transferred to all Kaiser Permanente regions. It includes the use of KP HealthConnect and
related electronic data systems and a wide-ranging toolkit of methods to notify eligible
members and to make it as easy and as convenient as possible for them to get their
mammograms. The campaign also focused on streamlining the steps between screening and diagnosis in order to dramatically shorten the number of "sleepless nights"
between a positive mammogram and follow-up biopsy and diagnosis.

Prior to Operation Innovation, women eligible for mammograms were identified
by an electronic database and were routinely notified by computer-generated letters
and by clinical staff during office visits. When these methods proved inadequate, a
series of more aggressive and personalized outreach and in-reach interventions was
designed by a multidisciplinary team of health professionals and specially trained
administrative staff. These steps included

- Improved electronic systems for identification of members eligible for mammograms;
- A robust telephone outreach to eligible members by specially trained call center staff;

- Personalized follow-up letters and telephone calls as needed by clinical supervisors;
- Use of a mobile mammography unit to reach members in underserved areas where mammography was not convenient or available; and
- "In-reach" by specially trained "welcoming committees" who greeted these patients when they arrived at the clinic for unrelated scheduled office visits. These members were offered immediate mammogram appointments during their visit.

In addition to these programs, cross-functional teams focused on increasing capacity and removing all barriers to timely and efficient interpretation of mammogram results, including creation of a special group of mammo-radiologists who excel at mammogram interpretation. This team also introduced new processes to dramatically shorten the time from suspicion of breast cancer to final diagnosis and surgical consultation.

The initial program achieved a dramatic increase in the percentage of eligible women receiving regular mammograms, rising from 79.5 percent at the inception of the program in December 2003 to 92 percent in January-February 2007. Major gains were also achieved in reducing the time from initial suspicion of breast cancer to diagnosis, falling from a median of nineteen days to nine days, with 79 percent of patients diagnosed within the target period of fourteen days.

By spreading these innovations across the regions and using KP HealthConnect to trigger reminders at every type of visit that a patient is due or overdue for a mammogram and linking directly to the mammogram reminder process, Kaiser Permanente in 2008 achieved the best breast cancer screening rates in the nation.

Central Venous Catheter Insertions. Patients who need frequent intravenous medication, blood, fluid replacement, or nutrition often have a tube or central venous catheter (CVC) placed into their veins, where it can remain for days and even weeks. However, CVCs can cause infections when bacteria grow in the catheter and spread into the patient's bloodstream, resulting in a catheter-related bloodstream infection (CRBSI). Each year, about 250,000 cases of CRBSI occur in hospitals throughout the United States, with an estimated mortality of 12 to 25 percent, or about 14,000 to 28,000 deaths annually (Centers for Disease Control and Prevention, 2002).

These central venous catheters are inserted into about one-half of all patients in intensive care units (ICUs), putting ICU patients at particular risk. For years, such infections had been accepted as an unavoidable problem, but that has changed. The Kaiser Permanente Sunnyside Medical Center ICU, in Clackamas, Oregon, has gone nearly three years with zero infections at the time of this writing—an achievement that would have been virtually unimaginable for any ICU just a few years ago.

Sunnyside physicians, ICU charge nurses, the IV team nurses, and infection control specialists teamed up to enable this transformation, with the help of KP HealthConnect. To begin, a group of quality-minded and evidence-based ICU physicians agreed to perform a "bundle" of multiple best-practice elements, based on guidelines from the Centers for Disease Control, when inserting CVCs. A key strategy was "to make the right thing to do the easy thing to do" for the physicians. Toward that end, a KP Health-Connect SmartTool was included, which requires the physicians to document performance of each aspect of the bundle in a checklist, thus both reinforcing knowledge of the bundle with each insertion and documenting adherence to the bundle for data collection purposes. IV team nurses who insert CVCs have a similar process for ensuring sterile insertion technique and universal adherence to the bundle.

After the CVC is inserted, meticulous ongoing catheter care is required to avoid infection. The Sunnyside ICU conducts daily, multidisciplinary ICU rounds that utilize a checklist that assesses if the CVC is still needed.

Sunnyside's remarkable success is due to physicians and nurses who understand that the overall quality of care depends on the reliable delivery of many small elements of care by different people at different times—a level of coordination almost impossible without IT support, which transforms best intentions into hard-wired excellence of care delivery.

Sunnyside's success in this area has provided confidence and a model for other quality improvement initiatives in the ICU, such as bundled measures aimed at reducing complications relating to invasive mechanical ventilation. KP HealthConnect is being reconfigured to once again make the right thing to do the easy thing to do. What is more, the Sunnyside success has set a high bar for ICUs throughout Kaiser Permanente, all of which are in pursuit of the same goal.[*]

Part Two: Proactive Care Management for Primary Care Physicians

Kaiser Permanente's selection of Epic System's electronic health record in 2002 was met with joy and elation in Kaiser Permanente's Northwest region, based in Portland, Oregon. The region had successfully piloted Epic's ambulatory medical record beginning in 1994 and had implemented it region-wide by the end of 1996. Instantaneous access to any patient's chart from anywhere in the region, combined with decision support at the point of care, had resulted in significant improvement in the region's quality performance. This demonstration of clinical excellence through medical

---

[*]Editor's note: The Sunnyside case study was contributed by David M. Schmidt, MD, Department of Pulmonary & Critical Care Medicine, and Dana Barron, RN, CIC Infection Prevention and Control Manager, Sunnyside Medical Center, Kaiser Permanente-Northwest.

informatics was acknowledged in 1998 when Kaiser Permanente-Northwest received the prestigious HIMSS Nicholas E. Davies Award of Excellence in implementation and value from health information technology, as well as Kaiser Permanente's own James A. Vohs Award for Quality.

At about this same time, Kaiser Permanente's Hawaii region was struggling with a series of EHR pilots. During these years, a group of dedicated Kaiser Permanente IT system managers and database analysts supporting both the Northwest and Hawaii regions had been mapping the extensive data flowing from the EHR and claims systems in each region into two regional data warehouses. The organization of this data was critical in creating the foundation of a population care infrastructure.

Population care experts in both regions mined this data to identify groups of patients with individual chronic conditions, creating registries for diseases such as diabetes, cardiovascular disease, asthma, and hypertension. Lists of patients with gaps in care were compiled for each primary care provider (PCP), printed, and mailed to them several times each year. Outdated and often inaccurate by the time they arrived, these lists became increasingly irrelevant and were often thrown away within days to weeks. The PCPs and their staffs were typically not given time to act on this information, as demands for access to office visits focused attention on the acute complaints that filled their schedules each day. Cancer prevention, chronic condition monitoring, and other important screenings occurred only when there was time. This was rarely accomplished reliably, especially when the patient's acute care needs dominated the vast majority of all encounters.

The implementation of KP HealthConnect across the program was expected to result in dramatic improvement in quality performance, including population care management. CEO George Halvorson boldly declared his goal of seeing each region achieve the 90th percentile on all HEDIS Effectiveness of Care measures. While no region was close to this level of performance at the time, the Northwest and Hawaii regions were further from this goal than most. Despite having instant access to extensive patient information and decision support at the point of care through the EHR for more than seven years, Kaiser Permanente's Northwest region was lagging in many quality measures. The EHR by itself hadn't been enough to achieve the level of superior performance that was now expected throughout Kaiser Permanente. It was going to take something more.

Many clinicians found that the additional coding and documentation requirements related to using an EHR took away time they had previously been spending with their patients. Desktop medicine meant clearing a never-ending stream of items such as lab results, staff messages, and patient phone calls from their in-baskets. Many PCPs complained that their practices and ultimately their careers were becoming unsustainable. The daily grind of providing reactive care to increasingly sick patients wore many of them down, leaving them exhausted by the end of their long clinic days. While the EHR allowed the clinician to focus more completely on each individual patient, very few had the energy to even think about the care needs of the entire population of patients they cared for—their panel. Many of their patients never came into the clinic and were effectively invisible to them. There had to be a better way.

Total Panel Ownership

In response to the shortcomings of the reactive primary care model, two primary care physician leaders from the Hawaii Permanente Medical Group, Jerry Livaudais and Samir Patel, developed a philosophy and system of proactive health care they described as Total Panel Ownership (TPO). TPO focuses on the PCP's relationship with members of his or her entire panel and also between the PCP and staff members—nurses, medical assistants, and others—supporting the practice. The team "owns" the health of the entire panel and commits to efficiently meeting their care needs, in part by empowering the support staff to work up to their full capabilities in staging this work for the clinician.

In the spring of 2005, Livaudais and Patel presented their TPO concept at the Institute for Healthcare Improvement (IHI) Summit on Clinic Redesign. They also called for the development of panel management technology that would allow care teams to not only assess the unmet care needs of each individual patient but also aggregate these care gaps, stratify them, and prioritize proactive care for the entire panel. Having met Livaudais and Patel at the conference, I shared their vision and decided to bring the TPO philosophy and care system to Kaiser Permanente's Northwest region by collaboratively building a panel management tool with Kaiser Permanente's Hawaii region. The tool was intended to support four Kaiser Permanente clinics that were participating in a primary care redesign project known as the 21st Century Care Innovation Project, described in Chapter Seven.

With $80,000 from the KP HealthConnect project and support from Kaiser Permanente's Care Management Institute, we met weekly via webinars with a small group of IT Web developers and database analysts to build the panel support tool (PST) by the end of 2005. The initial pilots in each region's first two clinics were very successful, and the findings were rapidly disseminated to other clinics. All of the adult primary care clinics in both regions had received up to ninety minutes of PST and Total Panel Ownership training by the end of 2006. Most clinicians had up to an hour of dedicated panel management time each day to enable patient outreach via phone, letter, or secure message, proactively meeting more of the needs of a larger population in non-visit-based encounters.

Managing the Entire Patient Panel

The Web-based, computerized member database is designed to complement KP HealthConnect. The tool allows PCPs and their staff to easily and proactively assess the health needs of individual patients or any cross-section of the panel without having to wait for analytic assistance. It then enables the provider to take needed action with the support of evidence-based systems of care. It is easy to use with little or no training, provides instant analysis, and enables immediate clinical action.

Every night, the PST downloads specific patient data from KP HealthConnect, the claims system, ancillary systems (lab, radiology, pharmacy), and the membership system and displays the information on a dynamic spreadsheet. It automatically sorts members with the highest care gaps to the top of the list of the patient panel. Care gaps are represented by numerical scores indicating the gap between recommended care and the care actually provided for each patient. For example, someone with coronary artery disease who has not filled a prescription for a statin or ACE inhibitor in the past six months, or has no documentation for aspirin use, would receive four points for each care gap. Patients are also stratified for disease severity, with color-coded information displayed for diabetes, cardiovascular disease, congestive heart failure, renal insufficiency, hypertension, asthma, and primary prevention (breast, cervical, and colorectal cancer screening, immunizations, blood pressure, osteoporosis, and lipids), as well as risk factors such as hyperlipidemia, obesity, and smoking. Pediatric content was added to the tool in early 2008 to support reliable delivery of well child visits, all childhood immunizations, and care for chronic conditions unique to pediatric practice.

Clinicians and their staffs can view and sort a broad range of conditions or other parameters, including preventive care needs, to identify widely prevalent gaps that might be addressed either one-at-a-time or many-at-a-time. Care gaps at the total panel or composite level can also be calculated for each panel for monitoring and assessing health improvement over time.

The most effective use of the panel support tool has resulted when the PCP is provided with sufficient dedicated time to monitor his or her panel and order appropriate actions. Another important condition is support from empowered and dedicated care team members who have the autonomy and freedom to innovate how care is delivered and to act proactively rather than only reactively. The complete care that is delivered by "max-packing" prevention and chronic condition management that wouldn't have otherwise been delivered in an exclusively problem-focused office visit has contributed to major improvements in quality performance in both regions.

Superior Quality Performance

As the shift to the total panel management approach has accelerated throughout Kaiser Permanente in recent years, several internal quality improvement studies have investigated various aspects of both the overall approach and use of the panel management tool itself. A 2006 internal study conducted in Kaiser Permanente's Hawaii region concluded that most physicians who had transitioned their practices to total panel management believed that the approach had improved the care they provide, especially to their more complex patients and their low-utilizing patients, who are otherwise rarely "touched" by the system. But they also noted that, despite having dedicated time for use of the tool to monitor their panel's health, the panel management approach added more tasks to their already busy days. As one PCP told investigators, "Panel management doesn't make my day any easier, but it makes my day better. It improves quality." In a 2008 survey of all Kaiser Permanente Northwest primary care clinicians, nurses and medical assistants, more than four hundred respondents (91 percent) reported using the PST to close care gaps for every patient, and 73 percent agreed "the PST has improved my work life."

Using KP HealthConnect and other key data sources, all eight Kaiser Permanente regions have implemented comprehensive panel management technology designed for front-line clinician and staff use. The reliable use of panel management support tools is producing superior quality performance, even when measured against the overall quality improvement seen among most major health plans.

Many regions are expanding their use of panel management technology beyond the primary care office to include other patient contact points, such as nurse treatment rooms and urgent care clinics. Several specialty care departments are also directing their medical assistants to use these tools to help their patients close care gaps reported by the panel management support tools during what is being called a "proactive office encounter." Future development of specialty-specific content for these tools will result in increased use and greater attention to prevention and screening. Specialty care departments in the Northwest region are currently looking for the first time at establishing secondary specialty panels to facilitate specialty support tool development. Successful panel management practices from each region are being adopted by other Kaiser Permanente regions, driving superior health outcomes, quality performance, and job satisfaction for physicians and staff across the program.

Part Three: Bringing Care Management to Specialty Groups

During the development of KP HealthConnect, clinical leaders came together from all regions to make shared decisions on how the system would support their practices. Although the initial purpose of these discussions was related to the development of clinical content for KP HealthConnect, the experience led to a continuing collaboration among leaders of various specialty groups related to broader issues, such as clinical goals, research priorities, and performance improvement. This in itself was a significant shift in clinical culture for Kaiser Permanente, where collaboration among the regions had long been desired but seldom optimized.

In primary care, the number of practitioners at Kaiser Permanente is in the thousands, and for these front-line physicians and nurses the organization purposefully funded development time for KP HealthConnect SmartTools and redesign of work processes, as discussed in Chapter Two. However, several of the Kaiser Permanente specialty groups found themselves facing the complex task of office reengineering for KP HealthConnect implementation with less IT support. In this section, we look at how some of these specialty groups, including practitioners in orthopedics, urology, and oncology, and a special interest group on domestic violence, harnessed the EHR to meet the needs of their patients and their practices.

Orthopedics and the Total Joint Replacement (TJR) Registry

Of the approximately 350 orthopedists within the Permanente Medical Groups, a small group emerged early on as eager adopters of KP HealthConnect. They readily took on the tasks of designing SmartTools for their common clinical situations and tamed the long lists of procedures and order sets on behalf of their colleagues. Whereas previously they had come together across regional lines for educational conferences and high-level interchange among their department chiefs, they now embarked on detailed reviews of work processes and clinical needs.

Thanks to the existence of common master files utilizing standardized medical terminology across all regional copies of KP HealthConnect, dedicated informatics-oriented orthopedists were able to develop tools for their entire specialty. They built, refined, and posted a variety of SmartTools on an intranet site and also put out educational tools to assist their less technology-adept colleagues in learning to use the tools. With help from the legal and regulatory staff in sorting out varying scope of practice requirements that existed across state jurisdictions, they were able to provide tools that took advantage of staffs' highest level of training and licensure.

Though the orthopedists varied in their prior use of electronic documentation tools, they were already sophisticated developers and users of data, as exemplified in the Kaiser Permanente Total Joint Replacement (TJR) registry. This registry began even before the full roll-out of KP HealthConnect and consisted of detailed clinical data on patients and devices used for total joint replacement (knees and hips), trauma management, ACL knee repair, and spine surgery. Thanks to work by the orthopedic chiefs, assisted by scientists and statisticians, we now have data on more than 75,000 joints registered, providing a vast amount of real-world information concerning different technical approaches to various surgeries and devices, matching patient characteristics to expected outcomes.

Orthopedists can now use features of KP HealthConnect to allow for easily performed functional status surveys of orthopedic patients at periodic intervals following surgery to better determine which procedures and devices are most effective for which patients. Data for the surveys can be gathered either during office encounters with patients or by "pushing" surveys out electronically to patients of various surgical cohorts through My Health Manager, the Web-based personal health record, at pre-specified intervals. They also enabled more automated data collection in the operating room and in the office through the use of barcoding functionality in the inpatient KP HealthConnect application and the use of SmartPhrase and SmartText in the ambulatory setting. Finally, they enabled enhanced data capture and analysis to help guide future practice by specifying a limited set of documentation choices.

One result of this work is that Kaiser Permanente now has the nation's largest and fastest-growing population-based TJR registry. Armed with data collected since 2001, Kaiser Permanente orthopedic surgeons can make more informed decisions about the most effective TJR implants and clinical practices. They are also able to better identify patients at higher risk of complications.

This kind of comprehensive, comparative data and analysis enables us to address one of the great deficiencies in American health care, which is the lack of good, evidence-based comparative information about what works. In Sweden, for instance, a national hip replacement registry has demonstrated a 50 percent reduction in surgical revision rates nationwide following identification and promotion of best practices among Swedish hip replacement surgeons. The revision rate in the United States, comparing Centers for Medicare and Medicaid Services data to the Swedish data, appears to be approximately twice as high as the rate in Sweden (Kurtz and others, 2007).

In orthopedics, new technologies come on the market frequently, but there has been insufficient tracking of their comparative effectiveness by independent parties to determine how well each new surgical procedure or device performs over time. The FDA, for instance, only requires device manufacturers to test their products against doing nothing, as opposed to alternative existing devices.

Without this information, orthopedic surgeons cannot identify best practices or recommend the most reliable implants. The use of less effective implants and surgical substances too often results in the need to do complete surgical revisions, a major burden for patients and a major contributor to spiraling total health care costs. Hip and knee total joint replacements, for example, are already the second highest cost for Medicare, and the overall annual cost is expected to rise to $65 billion per year by 2015 (Kurtz and others, 2007).

With the TJR registry and KP HealthConnect, we can now conduct, evaluate, and synthesize research into actionable clinical-care guidelines. One internal study, for instance, evaluated the best way to hold new joints in place. Manufacturer recommendations varied. Some patients had basic cement, some had hybrid surgical approaches plus cement, and some were uncemented. Until we evaluated the data, no one knew whether there was any difference in the survival time of the implanted joints based on the adhesive approach used.

FIGURE 6.1. SURVIVAL CURVES FOR CEMENTED, HYBRID, AND UNCEMENTED TOTAL KNEE ARTHROPLASTY.

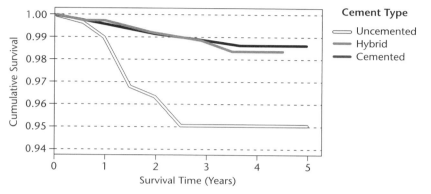

Analysis of registry data revealed a statistically significant difference in implant survival probability. Uncemented implants have lower survival probability compared with hybrid and cemented implants.

Analysis of the TJR registry data revealed there was a significant difference. The uncemented implants had a lower survival probability than either the hybrids or the cemented implants, as shown in Figure 6.1. In addition, registry data led to a reduction in the number of minimally invasive hip and knee procedures, which had promised, but did not deliver, reduced pain for patients. The data also resulted in practice changes with respect to implant selections when it was shown that certain new implant technologies were more costly than existing technologies, with no difference in outcomes (Paxton and others, 2008). When that data was shared across the organization, care practices changed and fewer patients ended up needing replacement implants. Data combined with shared learning made a difference in patient care (and the resulting cost of care) for the people who didn't need to have the surgery done twice.

Urology—Standardizing Evaluations and Reducing Radiation Risks

As with the orthopedists, the more than two hundred Permanente urologists constitute one of the largest single specialty practice groups in the country. For them, KP HealthConnect meant an opportunity to do focused, pragmatic research on areas of pressing concern. One of the most common referrals in outpatient urology is for asymptomatic micro-hematuria (painless blood in the urine). Our urologists estimated that, as a group, they saw more than 40,000 cases each year. But when they examined how they handled this clinical problem, they discovered wide variability in which patients were recommended for further invasive studies. Furthermore, they were becoming increasingly concerned about the amount of ionizing radiation that patients received with CT urography and were dissatisfied with the very low rate of actually finding serious genito-urinary disease and cancers. They saw the opportunity in KP HealthConnect to standardize their medical evaluations, track their data, and hone their approach to this common clinical condition.

In pursuing this quality improvement project, the urologists first commissioned an evidence review of the available scientific studies from Kaiser Permanente's Care Management Institute, which confirmed their suspicions that very little high-quality evidence existed to guide practice. So they worked across regions and asked our laboratories to consistently stratify and report hematuria. They then developed Smart-Tools that, as for their orthopedic colleagues, allowed for accurate, discrete, and consistent data in the EHR. Evaluation plans were also captured via standardized order sets, so that the positive results from diagnostic procedures such as cystoscopy and CT urography could be captured and analyzed.

However, standardizing the evaluations meant that potentially more patients would be sent for CT examination looking for tumors or kidney stones. In the light of recently published reports detailing the cancer risks of ionizing radiation, the urologists consulted with radiology colleagues to minimize patient risk. What followed was the development of a standard protocol for two-phase CT urograms, which reduced by one third the radiation incurred by the patients.

The results of this standardized evaluation are expected to drive further research in urinary cancer markers and establish new thresholds for hematuria requiring additional testing and evaluation.

Standardizing Protocols in Oncology

After the implementation and stabilization of KP HealthConnect, Kaiser Permanente became aware that the vendor, Epic Systems, was developing a new application for use in oncology. Assisted by specialty pharmacists and KP HealthConnect staff, we evaluated the functionality of the new product compared to home-grown systems already in use across Kaiser Permanente. While the existing systems were finely tuned to the needs of the oncology practitioners, the need to interface them with KP Health-Connect and the desirability of integrating the oncology treatment module into the clinical record proved to be a strong incentive for doing a national collaborative build of the Epic application for all of Kaiser Permanente.

An additional driving force was the increasing need to understand the practice patterns of oncologists, as cancer increasingly became the leading cause of death and as cancer drugs soared in cost. For the first time, we had the opportunity to understand the prescribing behaviors of our oncology clinicians, a feat that previous IT and pharmacy systems had not allowed. With the emergence of new quality measures being published by the American Society of Clinical Oncology, more insight into cancer treatment was imperative.

Under the leadership of the oncology chiefs and with one half-time, dedicated hematologist-oncologist, work was prioritized to address the most commonly utilized adult chemotherapy protocols, followed by those used in pediatrics, neuro- and gyn-oncology, and clinical trials support. Through frequent conference calls and the work of a dedicated oncology specialist pharmacist, the oncology chiefs group identified and standardized more than 230 protocols for the major adult cancers. Common nursing content was also developed and used across clinics. SmartTools were developed reflecting the protocols and physicians were able to enter the "intent"—curative or palliative—of the chemo regimen ordered. Thus linkage of protocols to subsequent clinical experience and complications of the patient enabled a better understanding of real-world practice outcomes than those from highly selected patients in randomized clinical trials.

The standardized protocols are meeting the bulk of clinical need, since they are being utilized over 80 percent of the time. In addition, new tools have been requested from Epic to facilitate the customization of protocols.

Once data is available from all oncologists, we will be able to feed data back to them to inform practice, as we have done with primary care for many years. We also hope that tools to easily identify patients who are eligible for experimental clinical trials will facilitate enrollment. In addition, metrics around efficiency in practice, such as infusion chair utilization, and safety metrics, such as use of alerts and analysis of possible adverse events, have been developed and are being used.

Since oncology medications are highly toxic, medication errors are of very serious concern. We wanted to be absolutely certain that the implementation of the EHR did not lead to unintentional harm. Therefore we monitored the number of medication errors in the first medical center to implement the new system before, during, and after the implementation, and were relieved to find no increase during implementation, and that errors decreased after implementation.

Screening and Treatment for Domestic Violence

The topic of domestic violence is not one commonly associated with the use of EHRs. Traditionally, many clinicians have been reluctant to even ask questions about domestic violence for fear the patient will respond in the affirmative, presenting the clinician with a challenging situation. An intense focus on this hidden clinical problem, which is a major cause of illness, injury, and death among women between the ages of eighteen and sixty-five, has resulted in a comprehensive, multidisciplinary program throughout Kaiser Permanente's Northern California region to screen health plan members, identify high-risk patients, and refer them to appropriate services within Kaiser Permanente and/or community-based programs.

The program, launched in a single service area in 1998 by Brigid McCaw, MD, MPH, now features clinical training in patient screening and identification for all primary care and specialty departments, Web-based treatment guidelines, and evidence-based screening and assessment tools embedded in KP HealthConnect (called the "DV SmartSet"). Other domestic violence best practices are distributed to clinicians via the KP HealthConnect SmartBook, discussed in Chapter Five. Extensive multilingual educational materials, including brochures, pocket cards, and resource information sheets are posted or otherwise available throughout the region's medical offices and a public Website (www.kp.org/domesticviolence).

Since the program was spread throughout the Northern California region, the number of Kaiser Permanente members identified as affected by domestic violence has increased three-fold, and, notably, most of the identifications have been made in primary care offices rather than emergency or urgent care departments, where victims typically appear following an actual injury. This suggests that at-risk individuals are being identified and offered counseling before they are injured.

This EHR-driven domestic violence program is now being implemented, in various forms, throughout all Kaiser Permanente regions. It has been nationally recognized as an innovative and model approach to a major but often unrecognized medical problem with awards from numerous national and local organizations for making a major difference in the lives of thousands of women and children.

EHR Implementation—Driving Care Re-Engineering

In each of these examples, a small subset of clinicians was able to develop standardized clinical content to achieve the goals of enhanced quality, research, efficiency in practice, safety, patient engagement, satisfaction, and consistent care—all leading to improved health care. Without the essential need to convene over the implementation and use of a common EHR, KP HealthConnect, it is unlikely that our clinicians would have had the opportunity to come together to do the detailed work of re-engineering their clinical work. And this is just the start of a long improvement journey. New functionality in each release of KP HealthConnect allows for different approaches to care and better alerting and decision support. New generations of clinicians are already comfortable and savvy with KP HealthConnect and are constantly looking to it for improvements in care and efficiency. Health care in 2015—just five years from now—will look as different from today's care as today's does from 2005.

CHAPTER SEVEN

REDESIGNING PRIMARY CARE WITH KP HEALTHCONNECT

By Ruth Brentari and Leslie Francis

Chapter Summary

This chapter describes a major initiative undertaken across Kaiser Permanente to redesign primary care practices in ways that could optimize the value of the electronic health record (EHR) while mitigating the new work demands associated with KP HealthConnect. The 21st Century Care Innovation Project proved effective in increasing various types of capacity in pilot sites, and many of the practice innovations that grew out of the initiative have been widely adopted. The chapter concludes with the perspectives and experiences of three primary care physicians who participated in the initiative and have continued leading efforts furthering this work well beyond the project.

Introduction

As the implementation schedule of Kaiser Permanente HealthConnect proceeded from region to region, concerns mounted about its impact on the workload and sustainability of the front-line primary care physicians who had been most impacted by

Ruth Brentari is senior director for Care and Service Quality; Leslie Francis is executive director in Kaiser Permanente's Office of the CFO.

the shift to an EHR and the attendant changes in workflow that came with it. In response, in 2005, in a partnership with the Institute for Healthcare Improvement (IHI), we launched the 21st Century Care Innovation Project, a pilot effort to transform primary care practices in ways that optimized the value realization of KP HealthConnect while addressing physician workload issues.

In some respects, these could have been competing goals. Tension existed between the organizational value of having an EHR and the additional stress that working with an EHR can place on physicians. While the impending primary care shortage wasn't as well documented in 2005 as it now is, we were aware that workforce adaptation to the technology was a key enabler to success. We also knew from past experience that optimizing KP HealthConnect to improve care delivery processes was not a passive journey. The project represented our belief that to realize value from KP HealthConnect for primary care, we needed to be explicit in our expectations, provide resources, and energize our care teams using the EHR to innovate.

Innovation Team Objectives

With the Blue Sky Vision for transforming care as framework, the objectives of the innovation project were to test new approaches to

- Deliver best health/health care outcomes to members;
- Deliver care that is more efficient and effective;
- Provide a superior care experience for members; and
- Promote a healthy and sustainable work environment for clinicians and staff.

Over the course of the project, we engaged a total of seventeen teams from five Kaiser Permanente regions and Group Health Cooperative of Puget Sound in Washington State. The teams consisted of a physician team lead, a clinic administrative lead, other practicing physicians, nurses, medical assistants, receptionists, and others such as nurse practitioners, analysts, KP HealthConnect staff, pharmacists, a project manager, and at least one patient member on each team. Project leadership was organized at the national level and worked with regional leaders accountable for primary care operations or quality.

The teams had broad boundaries for the innovations they could bring into the project. At the kick-off, they were encouraged to test a variety of changes as long as they were aligned with creating a new paradigm of health/health care delivery that could achieve the following objectives:

- Integrate and leverage KP HealthConnect to improve care delivery;
- Transform the delivery system to be patient-centered, as illustrated in Figure 7.1;

FIGURE 7.1. THE PATIENT-CENTRIC 21ST CENTURY CARE INNOVATION PROJECT MODEL.

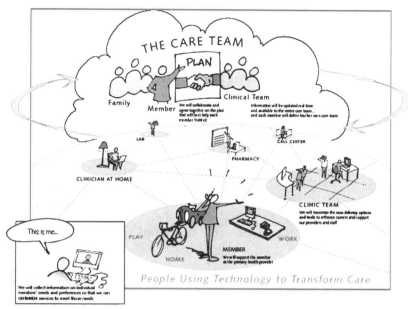

- Care for the member as a total being, not just a disease or condition;
- Empower members to be more proactive and engaged in their care;
- Create a process in which all members of the care team can participate in supporting the member's care—because information is available to all members of the team all the time; and
- Ensure that the work environment is sustainable and healthy for physicians and staff.

The Hypothesis—Building Capacity

What was consistent in the early months of the project was that the teams defined their work in terms of the practice's office appointment schedule. Their "line of sight" was today's and tomorrow's schedules. Access was an ongoing emphasis and challenge for most of the teams. Quality initiatives were tacked on as a task of the day and perceived as extra work. Short-term gains could be achieved, but it was difficult to sustain improvement. We needed to change that paradigm.

Our observation of the teams' work and the perspective of our two consultants, Chuck Kilo, MD, from Greenfield Health in Portland, Oregon, and Doug Eby, MD, from Southcentral Foundation in Alaska, led us to develop a hypothesis about the key process and people changes needed and how we could add value. The hypothesis was, if the teams designed the care team and their work to meet the needs of the population they were caring for (versus designing their work on the appointment schedule), and if they expanded the means by which they delivered care through phone visits, group visits, and ultimately e-visits, they could build capacity in the team using the same level of resources.

Furthermore, the team could use that new capacity to focus on the primary care physician's (PCP) panel of patients' unmet needs. We subsequently started referring to this expanded "line of sight" for the care team as "total panel ownership," a term borrowed from a primary care physician leader from the Hawaii Permanente Medical Group, Gerald Livaudais. We packaged the key work from the first innovation teams into a change package that we asked the teams to test more deeply, and in 2007 added several new teams to test the change package as a whole. The change package included the following concepts and process changes:

- Build the care team so that the team and workflows are organized to meet the needs of the population based on data. The care team as a whole must explicitly understand each member's role in meeting the needs of the population.
- Foster relationship-based care to create a patient-centered culture in which team members can say we really "know" our patients.
- Provide alternatives to 1:1, face-to-face visits to offer members options for receiving care.
- Practice Total Panel Ownership so that the PCP and team take care of all their patients' needs, as discussed in Chapter Six.
- Activate patients with collaborative care planning that empowers them to be the "real" PCP in the delivery system in making decisions and taking ownership of their own health.

KP HealthConnect, Panel Tools, and Innovation

KP HealthConnect functionality supported the teams' new workflows in several ways. For instance, unlike pre-EHR scheduled telephone visits, with KP HealthConnect all the relevant patient information is easily accessed by the provider during a phone visit. Real-time processing (notes, lab orders, prescription orders) is possible during a telephone visit. Work is completed during the telephone visit with few or no hand-offs required. Also, the Total Panel Ownership approach, described in Chapter Six, is supported by health maintenance alerts managed by the PCP's support team. The receptionist can schedule overdue screening appointments for patients without an order from the PCP, and medical assistants can transmit orders for the physicians that will satisfy care gaps for members with chronic care needs whenever they have an interaction with the member (for example, flu shot clinic). In addition, health maintenance information available to the care team is simultaneously available to the member via the member portal, My Health Manager. Finally, teams experimented with using KP HealthConnect's After Visit Summary to provide patients with documentation of their goals and personal action plans to reinforce collaborative care planning. Several teams tested sending electronic questionnaires to patients to capture key clinical signs or symptoms from the patients via secure e-messaging and to engage patients in their care at home.

Was the Hypothesis Proven?

Did we build capacity in the teams sufficiently to make sustainable improvements in quality and service? All regions experienced a drop in office visits with the implementation of KP HealthConnect. In addition, most of our pilot teams created additional capacity through the replacement of office visits with greater use of telephone visits and secure e-messaging. On average, teams experienced a 9 percent decrease in office visits per thousand members from the time they began the project, while overall provider contacts increased. The physicians in our first-year innovation teams saw on average 6 percent more of their panel of patients in the third year of the project than they did in the first.

In terms of quality performance, nearly all teams improved, with half outperforming their regions. Quality measures improved in the innovation teams faster than their regional counterparts, and several of the teams remain top-quality performers in their regions.

Our hypothesis about increases to member satisfaction levels was not proved conclusively during the project's duration. Most of the teams' overall satisfaction levels remained stable, although six teams improved at least 3 percent and some more than 10 percent in access satisfaction measures. In surveys, members rated the phone visits typically very high, similar to our office visit satisfaction ratings. In the very first year, work satisfaction improved for both physicians and staff, with physician work satisfaction improving more significantly.

Did we transform primary care? This first initiative showed the possibilities but did not demonstrate the full value of the investment. However, the objectives, the conceptual framework, and the change package have seeded innovative changes throughout the organization that continue today.

Physician Perspectives on EHR-Enabled Primary Care Redesign

In the following first-person accounts, three Kaiser Permanente primary care physicians relate their stories of primary care redesign set against the backdrop of the 21st Century Care Innovation Project and KP HealthConnect. The contributors represent different regions in the country, with different leadership accountabilities for various parts of their care delivery systems.

Backs Against the Wall in Hawaii

What drew me to participate in the innovation work? Quite simply, our backs were against the wall.

I was a part of a clinic with seven physicians serving a largely native Hawaiian population, many or most with chronic conditions. At first, KP HealthConnect was not seen as an aid to the clinicians. We all understood the value to the system at large, but as practicing physicians, we felt that it slowed us down and created more work. It is a significant paradigm shift for the clinicians. With a paper chart, you control to a certain extent the volume of work you do in a day. With an EHR, the sheer volume of clinical information that is available drives the workload. Let me paint a picture.

With the paper chart, I came in to the clinic in the morning and there was a stack of charts on my desk for the patients I would be seeing that day—lab and x-ray results to be reviewed, medication refills to consider and order. When I'd see my patients, completed my charts, reviewed the results, and signed the refills, my work for the day was done.

With the EHR, the work seemed never to be done. Now, if I am signing off on pharmacy refills, but 20 percent of those patients are due for preventive screening, I need to write the order for the screening tests and put the patient outreach call in place. If I am looking at a patient's chart for one reason and the system prompts me about a second care gap, I have to address that right away. The reality is that this isn't new work and it's always been there, but before the EHR it frankly was out of sight, out of mind. With KP HealthConnect, it's in your face, and any good clinician can't put it off.

It was clear we needed to make changes to take advantage of what the EHR offered to achieve better care and quality while simultaneously lessening the individual frustration levels.

Increased Capacity

Through involvement in the innovation work, we now believe we have increased our capacity—not just in the ability to handle the change the EHR brought, but in how my staff and I function as a team. We've created capacity in our "Plan, Do, Study, Act" skills, which has become our standard improvement paradigm; we've increased capacity to test new innovations and new technologies; and we've developed new capacity to let our members into our improvement process and learn directly from them. My day now starts with phone appointments with patients. I am an efficient problem solver and delegator, and I'm wired. I'm connected to KP HealthConnect and the member Web portal, our panel support tool, e-mail, secure instant messaging, and the phone. As I talk to a patient on the phone, I have the entire medical record in front of me at my fingertips and I "know" them. I document my assessment and plan as I would in an office visit; I order labs or change the medications; and I can do this from wherever the patient is comfortably speaking. While on the phone, I can also alert the patient about other care gaps they may have, for example, a mammogram or vaccine that is due. What's more, I can do "whole member care." If the patient and I decide that he or she needs to be seen in the office, the labs are ordered and often the results are in by the time the patient arrives at my medical office.

Before I start to see my office visit patients for the day, the entire clinic team (including doctors) attends a huddle. We quickly work through who needs help during the day and what each member of the team will focus on to take care of the panel, and we share data on a performance metric and reinforce the areas we need to improve. On my way back to my office from the huddle, I can see our "member council" going into the conference room for a meeting with our clinic leaders. These members/patients are becoming more empowered to make changes and give us feedback on how we are doing.

Caring for the Entire Panel

What is more, with the use of the phone, e-visits, and the panel tools, we have the capacity to look at and care for our entire panel of patients in real time. We identify those patients who are due for certain preventive interventions and can reach out to them automatically via phone or letter. We can now look at performance at a panel level and can involve the entire team in performance improvement conversations with this real-time data.

My care team has as much ownership for the care of my panel as I do. My medical assistant, for instance, prepares the charts for the patients we will be seeing in the office on that day, drafts orders to address care gaps identified by the panel tools, and does follow-up blood pressure checks on patients for whom I've changed their medication regime.

The innovation work forced us to rethink the work that we were doing, the roles each of the members of the care team played, and how they supported each other. It also made us realize that we weren't engaging one of the most important members of the care team—the patient and his or her family.

We have developed a real culture of innovation. We took on testing a new tool called the Archimedes Optimizer (see Chapter Eleven). This is a predictive model, using data from KP HealthConnect that provides individualized treatment recommendations to get the right treatment to the right patient. For my panel, for example, it predicts which patients will derive the most benefit from a given set of interventions or actions. Then for each individual patient, it provides a benefit score in a graph for each intervention. I use the visual display with the patient to prioritize together which interventions will have the greatest impact for them. We are really trying to push the envelope of patient engagement and collaborative care planning.

Getting Results

While the experience I've described is mine, it's also reflective of those of my colleagues and partners. Across the region, we now deliver 30 percent of our same-day care through phone visits—a major convenience to patients. By focusing on our panel of patients rather than the appointment schedule, we are producing better quality. Our region topped the national HEDIS rankings in breast cancer screening for 2008. We are using lean and Six Sigma methodologies, and we are mapping workflows and processes from "end to end" and hope to standardize them, while eliminating waste to help us with the next part of our journey.

We are still on our primary care redesign journey in Hawaii, and in some respects our backs are still against the wall. Four years ago we weren't certain what we could do that would help. Now, our challenge is putting all the things we have learned together in the right order with the right people in a way that adds value for our members, clinicians, and staff.

—Samir Patel, MD, assistant associate medical director, Kaiser Permanente-Hawaii

Strong Patient-Provider Connections Through Technology

I love challenges.

I lead primary care operations for 490,000 Colorado members, and we are fortunate in Colorado because we have become the employer of choice for primary care physicians coming from internal medicine and family practice training programs. The downside is that there are fewer and fewer who want those careers. At a time when it seems as though everyone is running away from primary care, I believe we have to lead our own physicians and staff to make it a better life and find a better way to practice.

We have created a path of process, staffing, and technology improvements that together are positioning us to deliver better care and better patient access to our physicians, and also a style of practice that is sustainable for the physicians. We believe a key to success is establishing and supporting the relationship between the physician and the member. In 2006, we implemented improvements to our panel management activities and focused on improving the ability of our members to routinely see their chosen PCP. By ensuring a reliable process for members to choose and see their primary physician we have improved our patient-physician "relationship" measure by 64 percent.

One of the challenges with primary care is sustaining your gains. There are always opportunities to improve. Two of our teams who participated in the 21st Century Care Innovation Project developed options for our patients that we believed would provide efficiencies for our members and also help us create capacity within the teams. In 2007 we implemented a telephony upgrade at our clinical call centers as well as scheduled telephone visits.

Scheduled Phone Visits

Scheduled telephone visits were another service option that we felt would improve patients' access to their physician. Without an EHR, the scheduled office visit was the trigger to get the paper medical record to the provider's office. With KP HealthConnect's immediate access to the patient's history, lab values, and problem list, our physicians could comfortably resolve many patients' questions over the phone.

We also introduced secure e-messaging for our members to connect with their physician and health care team. We currently respond to more than 30,000 secure e-messages a month in primary care, to the great satisfaction of our patients. We've leveraged the popularity of the scheduled phone and e-visits to re-implement advanced access to give our patients appointments when they want them. These alternative options gave the care teams additional tools to meet patients' needs. As a result, we have improved our administrative metrics of physician access by 66 percent, and these improved results are reflected in our satisfaction survey results directly from members.

We are now working on optimizing our care teams. With the primary care physician shortage looming, we believe we have to ensure that all of the members of our care team are working at their optimal scope of practice, and as a unit the care team and their workflows are designed to meet the needs of their panel of patients.

Our next improvement is to work on a system of engaging members in their own care. We are looking at the evidence for that work, trying to identify the keys to success in this area—there is considerable evidence on the value, but I don't believe anyone has yet found an effective design that is sustainable across physicians and care teams, over time. It will be a challenge.

—Scott Smith, MD, associate medical director, Kaiser Permanente-Colorado

Tactics for Transforming Primary Care

Was the deployment of Kaiser Permanente HealthConnect transformational in and of itself? It is clear that KP HealthConnect is an enabler, a tool, and a key decision-support ally in the day-to-day activities of a physician's work life. In my view, transformation of the Kaiser Permanente organization, as well as care delivery, is much more than the mere deployment and adoption of an EHR. But the dramatic change that is necessary would not be possible without the EHR.

Transformation in our organization implies a profound change in our structure, culture, and character while remaining true to our mission, vision, and core values, as well as our integrated strategy. Creating this transformational change is a large, complex, and challenging endeavor, given our ever-changing environment.

Underlying this transformation is the creation and adoption of a principled, consistent approach. I believe the centerpiece of this approach has been our senior regional leadership team. Highly visible, innovative, motivated, aligned, and not risk-averse, our team has demonstrated the capability of engaging the physician and ancillary workforces to help shape their capacity for meaningful change. Without this key ingredient, the transformation would not have been possible.

With the deployment of KP HealthConnect, our physicians and the organization sustained a significant disruptive impact to their work as well as their work-life balance. It was clear to me that more needed to be done to create a thriving work environment in order to balance the disruptive practice changes, physician autonomy, patient needs, and organizational requirements while augmenting quality, patient safety and satisfaction, and our global value proposition.

Keys to a Sustainable Work Environment

To meet that need, we commissioned and assembled a team of physicians, administrators, and our medical group board of directors. The end result was the creation of the Seven Tactics of Outpatient Care. These are

- Proactive office encounter;
- Proactive office support;
- Proactive panel management;
- Effective and efficient office management;
- Specialty physician role in primary care;
- Personal access and panel equilibration for adult primary care; and
- KP HealthConnect optimization.

We piloted a rapid cycle improvement process for the refinement of each tactic at several medical offices. Once identified as a mature, deployable initiative, these operational imperatives were exported throughout our 150 medical office buildings and twelve Medical Centers.

Our earliest transformational tactic, the proactive office encounter (POE), is key to the creation of a highly reliable, reproducible, clinical approach to proactively identify care gaps during a face-to-face encounter in any primary or specialty care department. By leveraging KP HealthConnect along with related online clinical tools, including our disease registry and decision-support engine, we have accomplished much to change the course of care and the lives of millions of patients.

The benefits are clear in our improved screening rates for breast cancer, cervical cancer, hypertension control, monitoring HbA1c, and colorectal cancer, all of which are among the highest in the organization. In addition, the POE has enabled us to avoid 100,000 unneeded cervical cancer screening appointments. Even more impressive, it has allowed us to reduce stage four colorectal cancers at the time of discovery by 26 percent, ensuring greater survival rates. It has improved quality, affordability, and patient safety and satisfaction scores; reduced waste; and improved patient accessibility.

Value of Data Mining

All of our tactics are supported by analysis of the data from KP HealthConnect. In fact, I believe the data-mining opportunity will be the single most important value of the EHR over time. Because of our scale, KP HealthConnect data mining is currently a resource-intensive effort and requires skilled programmers working in support of physicians and operational leaders. Despite those hurdles, we are continually improving on the availability of KP HealthConnect information to support decisions on enhancements to our daily operations, physician proficiency with KP HealthConnect, and analysis of our care delivery patterns.

During the next phase of our care delivery transformation, we will leverage our integrated care delivery system, enabled by KP HealthConnect, with the aim of becoming the national leaders in preventive care, chronic disease management, cancer detection and its treatment, creating the safest hospitals in the United States, and providing the most robust care options for end-of-life care in the country.

In summary, the IT-enabled transformation of an integrated care delivery system is complex, arduous, and filled with unexpected findings. In the end, enhancing our organizational value requires explicit delivery system changes, multiple initiatives, and engaged organizational leadership to execute this change.

—Paul Minardi, MD, medical director for Operations, Kaiser Permanente-Southern California

CHAPTER EIGHT

MAKING HEALTH PERSONAL

By Kate Christensen, MD, and Anna-Lisa Silvestre

Chapter Summary

Kaiser Permanente's early development of the electronic health record intersected with separate initiatives for using the Internet and the Web to improve member service and patient care. The convergence of these efforts was to add significant new functionality and value to the EHR by providing an online portal through which members and patients could directly access their medical records and a variety of online health tools and information. This chapter discusses the challenges of that convergence and how the organization and its members are now realizing the benefits of the nation's most widely used personal health record.

Introduction and Background

Like many companies in the early days of the Internet, Kaiser Permanente began exploring the rapidly evolving new digital communication technologies for how they might improve the delivery of services to our customers—our members and patients—not knowing where it might lead. In the early 1990s, we anticipated that

Kate Christensen, MD, is medical director, Internet Services Group; and Anna-Lisa Silvestre is vice president for Online Services, both in Kaiser Permanente's national office. Judy Derman and Jan Oldenburg also contributed to this chapter.

the path we were embarking on could intersect with the simultaneous initiatives in various Kaiser Permanente regions to develop EHRs.

In our Northern California region, a handful of inquisitive people with backgrounds in member health education were looking at how the new interactive technologies could be used to connect the health system with its members in nontraditional ways. This early group focused on cable modems, kiosks, CD-ROMs, and various software products and asked, "What is it that we could be doing with these new tools?" The group included physicians, nurses, technologists, and other staff across the region. Together, led by Tim Kieschnick, they wrote a forty-page white paper proposing an overall strategy to explore the potential uses of new media and technology, especially in the areas of decision-support tools for members, clinical medicine (telemedicine and remote consultation), psychosocial support for patients, and member business functions. This work resulted in the funding of the Interactive Technology Initiative (ITI) as a small research and development effort and the appointment of Anna-Lisa Silvestre as the ITI business manager.

It was at about this time, in the mid-1990s, that the World Wide Web exploded upon the Internet as a new and compelling communication tool with the commercialization of the Netscape browser and its graphical user interface. As the Web grew exponentially, the ITI group refocused its work exclusively on developing a Website for Kaiser Permanente members that would have basic health education and limited interactive functionality.

Netscape was hired to build the first Website, which was deployed in 1996 and offered to just a thousand Kaiser Permanente members who used the Santa Clara Medical Center, in the heart of California's Silicon Valley. The project's sponsor was Robert Pearl, MD, the executive medical director and CEO of The Permanente Medical Group in Northern California. The first server for the Website was housed on little more than a card table in a Kaiser Permanente office. It was some months before the number of registered users reached even a hundred. The site featured online discussion groups, medical facility directories, a health encyclopedia, an online advice nurse feature, and the ability to book some nonurgent appointments.

The following year, the group overseeing the site, christened KP Online, was moved into Kaiser Permanente's national offices in Oakland, and the infrastructure was significantly enhanced by installation of a robust server at the Kaiser Permanente data center in Silver Spring, Maryland, capable of supporting the roll-out of the site across the entire national organization. At that time, in 1999, we had approximately 117,000 KP Online users, who registered through a somewhat clunky two-step process. First, they entered their member identification information on the Website, and then an authentication code was mailed to their address of record. They then entered the code on the Website and chose a password. Many found this process cumbersome—a problem that took several years to resolve with a streamlined, one-visit process.

As is common with radically new technologies, the first design of the Website copied the world we knew and had category names like Bookshelf and Classroom, taken straight from the health education departments in the medical centers. Soon after going live, it became clear that users were having trouble finding what they needed. On the basis of formal usability testing with users, the site was completely redesigned, and ever since then every new enhancement of the site has been tested with users from the very beginning.

By this time, Kaiser Permanente was moving forward with a planned organization-wide EHR—the predecessor of KP HealthConnect—and teams from both the EHR initiative and KP Online were planning for how clinical data from the medical record could be shared with members via the Website. Alan Eshleman, MD, the first physician on the KP Online team, had an inkling of the potential impact of giving patients a window into their electronic health records, noting in a journal article in 2000 that "the impact of the (solutions) we develop will be as transforming for clinical medicine as the telephone was in the late 19th century—perhaps even more so, because the Internet has grown explosively over a much shorter period than the telephone did" (Eshleman, 2001, p. 78).

In 1999, the original members-only Website was merged into the organization's public site, kp.org, making all of KP Online's nonsecure information, such as facility directories and the health encyclopedia, which did not require a password to access, available to the public, while access to all the secure, member-only functions, such as appointment scheduling or e-messaging doctors, remained password-protected.

By 2009, the group overseeing Kaiser Permanente's Websites, now known as the Internet Services Group (ISG), had grown from a handful of health educators to a large, national department of more than two hundred professionals, and the obscure little Website with a hundred users had become an integral part of one of the nation's most sophisticated online care delivery system, serving more than three million registered users. Kp.org had become a game changer in health care delivery.

Creating a Patient Portal into the EHR

With the adoption of the Epic software and implementation of KP HealthConnect, as described in earlier chapters, new opportunities arose in 2003 to provide Kaiser Permanente's members with direct Web-based access to their medical records, using the Epic module called MyChart.

At the time, the password-protected section of the kp.org Website already had an established presence for a growing number of members. For the ISG, the design challenge was to incorporate this new capability—the online health record—into the existing site with a minimum of disruption. This was accomplished by adding "tiles" or special iFrame Web pages that gave patients a view into their medical records from within the existing Website. As a result, members have an integrated experience, with all the separate parts working in concert to help users easily complete their health-related tasks. This kind of medical record access is quite different from systems that offer only an extract of patient clinical information based on claims data, which may or may not be complete. Registered kp.org users can see the most important parts of their actual health record—the same record their doctors use.

Beginning in mid-2005 in Hawaii and concluding in late 2007 in California, the MyChart window into members' medical records—renamed My Health Manager—was made available to all 8.6 million Kaiser Permanente members across the nation. The features included test results, allergies, diagnoses, immunizations, prescription lists, summaries of past office visits, secure messaging, and proxy access (the ability to act for a family member). Since then, the regions have continued to add features.

As the roll-out was proceeding, a Total Health Assessment tool from Health Media International was added in 2006, with a set of online self-management programs for problems such as back pain, insomnia, stress, weight, and smoking. Woven into many of the terms displayed on the online health record are links to topic pages in the Website's Health Encyclopedia (from HealthWise) and Drug Encyclopedia (from First DataBank) that explain the diagnosis, drug, or test in lay language, much of it also available in Spanish.

Regional Roll-Outs

In a multiregional organization such as Kaiser Permanente, the roll-out of any new technology or program must address the different needs, capabilities, and priorities for each region. As with the roll-out of KP HealthConnect itself, collaborative decision making between and among the national offices and the regions was the order of the day in deploying the online medical record.

In the roll-out phase, an important milestone was a series of planning meetings with front-line staff and physicians to discuss what technical changes a region could make to any particular feature and what the operational implications would be. These sessions were crucial to obtaining regional buy-in and support. Physicians, nurses, medical assistants, administrators, labor representatives, call center agents, and compliance staff, as well as representatives from other stakeholder groups, attended these regional sessions to resolve such issues as What types of appointments could members schedule and cancel online? How would the members' messages be securely routed? How would members notify their physician if they thought something in their online record was incorrect?

Communication and training were also important aspects of preparing for the implementation of the online record access in the regions. A number of the regions developed online and/or in-person training by implementation teams for physicians and other clinicians to learn technical skills such as using the member messaging functionality and releasing lab results for member access. Even more important was training on how to use kp.org to enhance their relationship with patients.

Principles Governing Patients' Health Data Access

As one set of teams worked on the complex technical task of creating this integrated and secure online experience, another laid the policy foundation for the work by articulating the principles that would guide specific decisions about access to personal health data. This work was led by the Website medical director, Kate Christensen, MD, who continues to provide oversight and leadership for all the clinical aspects of kp.org. These principles are consistency, accessibility, security, and transparency. They are all based on the patient-centered, home-is-the-hub perspective that came out of the original Blue Sky Vision, described in Chapter One.

Consistency. Consistency regarding access to the health record was a foundational principle, based on fairness or justice. Some health care systems with EHRs allow each physician to decide which patients have electronic access to their record and which are allowed to send them e-messages. In addition to being inequitable, such an approach overlooks the fact that the ability to access one's health record is not just a convenience but an important tool in equipping patients to be active participants in their own care. Consistent application of access rules across entire patient populations is not only fair, it is better care.

Accessibility. The principle of accessibility is also based on fairness. The kp.org Website seeks to provide online health record access to all Kaiser Permanente members who want it. We are much of the way there, providing access to all capable adults, to incapacitated adults via an approved proxy, and to children under twelve or thirteen (the age varies by state) via their parents or other care givers. Teens are a difficult group to deal with because of the complex and inconsistent privacy laws that vary by age, condition, treatment, and state. We are continuing to explore ways to create meaningful and useful access for teens and, when appropriate, their parents.

Security. Most people who use a health Website that involves their personal health information assume that the site is secure, and Kaiser Permanente goes to great lengths to ensure that it is. Kp.org adheres to industry standards for security and performs ongoing security testing to make sure all processes are up to date. The organization's privacy policy, as well as its Code of Ethics, is posted prominently on the Website. Kaiser Permanente's policy is to not share members' personal information without their explicit permission. In no circumstances does Kaiser Permanente sell member information, and the site does not host any advertising.

Transparency. Transparency is a watchword now in government and business, but in health care it has been a controversial term at times, especially as regards patient access to the medical record. Some health care organizations give physicians individual discretion about which diagnoses or tests a patient is allowed to see online, blocking access to any results or conditions that the physician feels might make the patient uncomfortable or frightened, or could create misunderstanding. But viewed from the patients' perspective, this approach can leave them wondering, "Why are some of my tests available and others not?" "Why isn't my irritable bowel syndrome listed as a condition, when I've seen the doctor for it four times this year?" "Is there something wrong she's not telling me about?" "Don't they have complete records on me?" "Is there something wrong with their system?"

From a philosophical or legal perspective, all of the data in the patient's chart originates with the patient—it is their blood and urine, their lungs being x-rayed, their blood pressure that is too high or too low. In fact, the patient already has the legal right, guaranteed by the 1996 Federal Health Insurance Portability and Accountability Act (HIPAA), to a copy of their medical record, although the usual paper version is rarely convenient to obtain or read, nor is it free (in the old days, patients often had to obtain a subpoena to see their medical record). For all these reasons, Kaiser Permanente established from the beginning that we would make online access to the record as complete as we could—within the limits of the law—while avoiding predictable harm to the patient. In California, for instance, state law prohibits electronically showing patients test results that might show drug abuse, cancer, HIV status, or infectious hepatitis.

Despite some legal limitations, patients' access to their medical information is significant. For instance, in our Colorado region the patient can access some test results as soon as they are available to the doctor, sometimes within hours, including cholesterol panels, hemoglobin A1C (a test for diabetes control), strep tests, influenza tests, and pregnancy tests. The results of other tests are accessible after forty-eight hours, including acute hepatitis panels, TB tests, drug and alcohol levels, most kidney and liver tests, most metabolic tests, allergy tests, chemistry tests, and urinalysis. A few complex test results are not accessible for seven days, including tumor markers and genetic testing. This delay allows the physician a chance to talk with the patient about the results, but if that does not occur within seven days, the patient can access his or her results.

While unmediated access to certain kinds of test results is less than ideal, we believe this serves as an additional safety net to ensure that test results are communicated to the patient. The need for such a safety net was shown by a 2009 study that reviewed the medical records of more than 5,400 non-Kaiser Permanente primary care patients. It found that the average rate of failure to inform or to document informing patients of clinically significant test results was more than 7 percent (Casalino and others, 2009). When millions of lab tests are performed every month, 7 percent can be a very big number. Providing the results directly to patients can help prevent delayed diagnoses and limit the anxiety of waiting for a test result.

Some diagnoses are blocked from member access in kp.org to prevent patient harm, in particular those related to domestic or child abuse. The intent is to ensure that an abuser would not be able to see the online record "over the shoulder" of a patient who sought care for abuse, potentially risking further abuse as a result. Similarly, abuse diagnoses are not disclosed on appointment slips and other notifications to the patient, for the same reason. Other diagnoses have been slightly modified so that they would be understandable to patients, such as "history of neuroendocrine cancer" instead of "HX of neuroendocrine CA." When the clinical term is retained, patients see the same terms they see when the doctor shares the KP HealthConnect screen with them during an office visit, and they will also be better able to research their condition online, look for clinical trials, and join in online support groups.

One area of particular concern is related to patients' access to their mental health diagnoses. The fear is that patients might be harmed by seeing diagnoses of depression, anxiety, schizophrenia, or bipolar disease. A group of Kaiser Permanente mental health leaders established a policy that clinicians need to talk to patients frankly about their mental conditions and the basis for their diagnoses. Showing the clinical diagnosis online could motivate reluctant clinicians to engage in such discussions, and would also help patients use accurate clinical terminology to search for online information about their conditions. The one exception was for the diagnosis of paranoid psychosis, which can be referred to online simply as "mental health disorder" to avoid potentially harmful patient reactions.

Listening to Member Input. As noted earlier, each of these principles is directly related to the overriding framework of patient-centered health care. Members are provided online access to their actual health records because it empowers patients to be better informed and equipped to participate in their care as partners with their physicians. In support of this framework, every effort has been made to make kp.org work for members, and that has meant working *with* members. From the very beginning, starting with user testing, surveys, and focus groups, the voice of members and patients has been critical to the success of kp.org. A formal in-person Member Advisory Panel meets periodically to serve as a sounding board and think tank for existing features and possible enhancements, and member input has been recently expanded to include a large virtual advisory group, with more than 30,000 participants.

Clinical Oversight. Along with member input, the active and deep participation of physicians from throughout the organization has been essential to creating an online care tool that enhances and supports the vital patient-physician interaction. Physicians routinely review all kp.org health articles and provide input on priorities and feature enhancements. The Internet Services Group health team created a formal Clinical Advisory Group, including physicians, nurses, and organized labor partners. This group tackled the difficult recommendations for test result access and diagnosis display, along with myriad other clinical recommendations.

Through this process of careful user testing, surveys, focus groups, and member and clinician advisory groups, a set of recommended settings for each feature was developed as the national recommendation to all Kaiser Permanente regions, which then weighed in with their own decision-making processes and priorities. What emerged was a set of online capabilities that guaranteed consistency, accessibility, security, and transparency for all users while being adaptable to the unique needs of each region when necessary.

Building Stronger Patient-Physician Relationships Online

The electronic health record and patient secure messaging are helpful beyond just the daily practical tasks of refilling medications and reviewing lab tests. These are time-saving tools that also help me to deliver better care and build patient relationships. A woman patient of mine was very distressed about her worsening hair loss. She had scheduled a nonurgent clinic appointment online, but it was some weeks away. We were able to work through it together through kp.org, eliminating systemic causes by ordering appropriate lab tests, reviewing recent medications, and starting some preliminary treatment before I saw her in the clinic. We discussed her recent emotional stresses, and I offered her support. By the time she came for her clinic visit, we had eliminated several potential causes and were able to quickly proceed to the exam, confirming our working diagnosis. Through encounters like this, I have become more responsive to individual needs and have forged better relationships with my patients. At the end of the day, I am less frustrated and can feel good about the care I can provide for my patients.

—Cynthia Mates, dermatologist, Kaiser Permanente-Northern California

Adoption and Usage

The public's perceived lack of engagement with online health records, referred to as "personal health records" (PHRs), has been the subject of considerable debate within the industry about why the adoption rate has so far been low and what the public really wants in a PHR (Kahn, Aulakh, and Bosworth, 2009). According to some estimates, only about 3.5 percent of consumers were using PHRs by early 2009 (Moore, 2009).

We believe the surveys have been asking the wrong question. Kaiser Permanente's own experience with My Health Manager is that consumers will adopt online health services on the basis of perceived usefulness and perceived quality. They want to e-mail their doctors, see their lab test results, view summaries of their office visits, and make appointments online. Kaiser Permanente data indicates that our members across the age continuum are adopting online health tools, and that usage spans income levels (Silvestre and others, 2009).

My Health Manager Registrations

As of September 2009, kp.org's My Health Manager continued to be the most widely used PHR of its kind, with the total number of registered patients hitting 3.3 million (see Figure 8.1). Excluding members under the age of thirteen and those without access to the Internet, the adoption rate was 63 percent of Kaiser Permanente's total membership, and an additional 80,000 new users, on average, registered each month.

Once members register and visit the site, most of them return: in 2008, 54 percent of users accessed My Health Manager five or more times. The kp.org site logs in more than five million visits per month, and more than 96 percent of those are to My Health Manager. Daily visits to My Health Manager averaged approximately 72,000, an increase of more than 18 percent from January to September, 2009, and the number of unique visitors (separate individual users) increased more than 17 percent. Not surprisingly, the majority of users (58.7 percent) are female, and a similar majority (57.3 percent) is between the ages of thirty-six and sixty-five. Despite preconceptions to the contrary, about 48 percent of all members age sixty-five and older were registered users.

Making the registration process as easy as possible was an important key to increasing the return rate. As noted earlier, the initial registration procedure involved a two-step process, which resulted in completion rate of only 60 percent. In 2008, a new one-step online identity verification process, widely used in the financial industry, was

FIGURE. 8.1. MY HEALTH MANAGER MEMBER REGISTRATIONS, JANUARY 2007–MAY 2009.

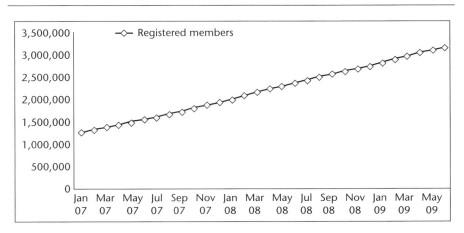

introduced, and the completion rate increased to approximately 90 percent. Members can also still opt to have the activation code mailed to their home address rather than answer online ID verification questions.

My Health Manager's high adoption rate is attributable to the perceived usefulness of the service. Compared to stand-alone PHRs, which are not linked directly to providers' clinical records, My Health Manager provides a direct link to the patients' clinical records and to their physicians. The data it contains is not self-populated by the members, with inevitable gaps and inaccuracies, nor is it derived solely from insurance claims data. My Health Manager accesses the same clinical data that is entered by and used by their health care providers, which means it is complete, accurate, and up to date. In addition, it is linked to the online medical staff directory, with extensive information about physicians, including photos, biographies, credentials, training, and languages spoken. This makes it easy to research and choose a physician, or to change doctors if desired.

Most Visited Features

Test Results. The "View My Test Results" feature on My Health Manager was an instant success from the beginning, and usage has been climbing steadily, as shown in Figure 8.2. Kaiser Permanente members were viewing an average of 5.2 million test results every month as of August 2009, for a total of more than 42 million since the feature was first launched.

FIGURE 8.2. STEADILY INCREASING USAGE OF "VIEW MY TEST RESULTS."

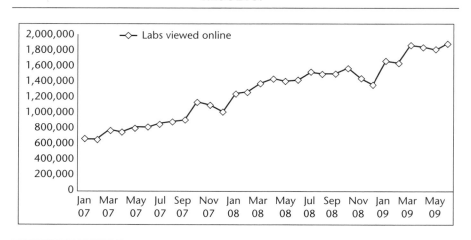

The vast majority of these results were released automatically. For example, from January to August 2008, more than thirty-seven million test results were released automatically, without the intervention of a physician. Of those, a small percentage were released on a time delay, from two to seven days, depending on the region and type of test, and the remainder was released manually by the physicians from within the electronic health record, often including a note to the patient regarding the result.

E-mail Your Doctor. The "E-mail Your Doctor" feature rapidly became one of the most popular functions. More than eighteen million secure messages have been sent since the feature debuted in 2005, and by May 2009 an average of 361,000 members were sending a total of 700,000 e-messages to their providers every month, as shown in Figure 8.3.

The popularity of the provider e-messaging function is just one of many influences on patient satisfaction, cost savings, and overall care quality. But there is emerging evidence that it has contributed to a decrease in patient office visits and telephone contact rates. A 2007 study examined the use of secure e-messages between Kaiser Permanente members and physicians. Patients with online access to their electronic health record were 7 to 10 percent less likely to schedule an office visit and made about 14 percent fewer phone contacts than those not using the online services (Zhou and others, 2007).

FIGURE 8.3. NUMBER OF MONTHLY MEMBER E-MESSAGES TO PROVIDERS, JANUARY 2007–MAY 2009.

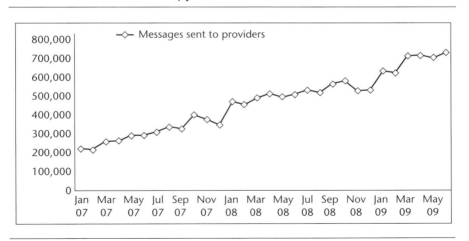

Another indication of the positive impact of the e-messaging feature emerged from the disastrous southern California wildfires in October 2007. For days at a time, Kaiser Permanente medical offices in the San Diego area were open or closed depending on the threat of nearby fires and wind conditions. With secure e-mail messaging, members who could not see their physicians directly were nonetheless able to communicate with them and thus to manage certain health conditions or other medical issues online. E-mail messaging to providers during that month increased by 35 percent, from 34,500 to 46,000.

Online Rx Refills. Another consistent favorite is the online refill request feature, which was generating almost 600,000 requests a month as of May 2009 (see Figure 8.4). Members can request refills for themselves or their family members (with privacy safeguards), elect to have any co-pay charged on their credit card, and pick up the medication or have it mailed to their home without an extra charge. Not surprisingly, more than 60 percent of refills are mailed to members' homes. This feature saves members time and inconvenience and is more efficient for the Kaiser Permanente pharmacies, as well. It is also possible that the convenience of online refill requests and home mailing leads to better adherence to medication regimens and thus to better health outcomes—a subject for future study.

FIGURE 8.4. MONTHLY ONLINE PRESCRIPTION REFILL REQUESTS, JANUARY 2007–MAY 2009.

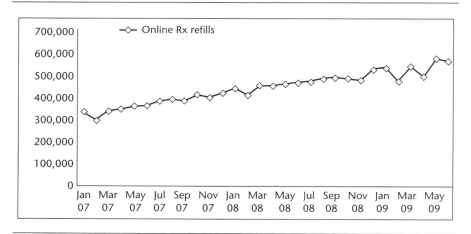

Special Issues

Following are some of the major issues, challenges, and unresolved questions that will inevitably arise in the course of creating and managing online patient access to an EHR.

Incident Management

One thing that is certain is that there will be incidents to manage: Website or feature outages; misuse of passwords to access another individual's health information; users not recognizing their own data online because they do not recognize the name of the physician; confusion created when patients have shared e-mail addresses; parental disputes related to proxy access to a child's health information. To deal with these types of urgent problems, we created a dedicated incident team with staff available 24/7 to rapidly investigate and either solve incidents or refer them to the appropriate organizational group, such as a compliance officer or customer service. Reviewing and tracking incidents is an important source of data for improving the Website functionality.

Acting for a Family Member

From the beginning of the development of My Health Manager, the Kaiser Permanente team planned to develop the capability for members to take appropriate action on behalf of a family member. For example, we wanted to empower parents to be able to communicate with their children's doctors and easily obtain immunization records for camp or school enrollment. We also wanted to enable adult children to be able to understand their parents' medical care, and to enable spouses to act on one another's behalf. Furthermore, we wanted a convenient way for members to sign up for such approved access without requiring them to be present in person. The legal and policy implications of developing and implementing this capability turned out to be more profound and complex than anyone anticipated.

One of the first questions we needed to answer was how we would know that someone was a family member of the patient in question and that the person was authorized to act on their behalf. For children under the age of twelve or thirteen (exact age is determined by state law), parents or guardians needed to apply for access to their children's records. If the applicant's address of record is the same as the child's in the Kaiser Permanente membership database, the person is provided with immediate online access; if the applicant lives at a different address than the child, the parent's password is sent to the child's address. Adults who apply for access to a child's record electronically sign an attestation that they are entitled to have access to the child's record. The attestation must be repeated every two years, and the parental access expires when the child turns the age specified by the state.

Similar functionality was launched to enable adults to access the records of other adults in 2008. The key difference between the capabilities for adults and those for parents is that in adult-adult access, the person who owns the account needs to give permission (from their secure account in kp.org) for the other person to have access to the account. Those permissions need to be renewed every two years. This approach enables adults to choose who they want to have access to their health record online, enabling them to create a circle of caring friends and relatives to suit their needs. The following e-mail message to a Kaiser Permanente physician from a patient offers a clear example of how valuable such proxy access can be for elderly spouses.

> Dear Dr. _____
>
> I would like to encourage you to keep using kp.org. Since I have started communicating with you via the Internet it is so much easier to get instructions from you concerning George's health and how to care for him. It's especially good to be able to read changes in medication dosages, that way I make a copy and have it at hand when I need it.
>
> Your concern for our well-being is surely appreciated, and using kp.org makes us so comfortable in communicating with you. . . . George has so much confidence in you and when he's feeling bad he tells me to e-mail you and you will take care of him. Thank you for that.
>
> Please continue using kp.org.
>
> Thank you.
> A Kaiser Permanente
> patient (name withheld)

Clinician Concerns

As expected, many clinicians were initially concerned that their patients were not ready to see their actual health data without the physician acting as an interpreter and intermediary. Although patients have long had a legal right to obtain most of their medical record, there were logistical and economic obstacles that made it unlikely that patients would do so, except for a specific legal or medical need. For physicians, the medical record was always where they communicated with other clinicians about the patient, and not always in a way that a lay person might understand. Lab test and radiology interpretations were usually written in the shorthand, jargon, and abbreviations essential to efficient communication among similar professionals. For example,

"SOB" written in a chart means "short of breath," but could easily be misunderstood by a patient. Nothing in the medical record was ever written with the thought that the patient could be reading it the next day. The prospect that patients could now access parts of their record at the click of a mouse, at any time, was naturally unsettling to many physicians.

Most of these concerns were resolved through extensive discussion and communication among the concerned physicians and medical group leaders, and reinforced through their own experience with patient access to the EHR. Many of the strongest critics became, over time, the strongest champions of online health record access. Fears that patients would react anxiously or inappropriately to seeing their test results have proven largely unfounded. Patients have now viewed millions of test results, with only a handful of complaints, and with high satisfaction levels.

Implementing Twenty-First Century Health Care

In the twentieth century, quality medical care, access, and affordability were viewed as trade-offs. In the twenty-first century, thanks to advancements in modern technology, it is possible to provide all three.

The office and hospital-based electronic health record allows physicians, nurses, and other clinicians to treat patients more rapidly, maximize patient safety, and achieve superior quality outcomes. Having the totality of clinical information immediately available, physicians can take a comprehensive approach to care delivery, follow clinical expert-recommended approaches to care, and eliminate redundant testing and interventions. Illness can be prevented, complications can be avoided, and treatment of life-threatening illnesses facilitated to an extent not previously imagined. The combination of a comprehensive electronic health record with sophisticated Internet-based tools allows health care to move from episodic to continuous care and to be available wherever the patient may be.

When physicians and other clinicians experience the degree to which advanced IT systems enhance the medical care they provide to their patients, they embrace the technology. However, implementation and the successful integration of the technology into clinical practice require physician leadership. Leaders must ensure that clinicians understand why change is required, how they will be supported in the transition, and the improvements in health outcomes that will result. Providing the highest quality care in the most professionally satisfying way is what motivates physicians and others in health care. Helping to translate this vision and potential into practice is the role of physician leadership. When it is done well, clinicians enthusiastically embrace the new capabilities that exist. As evidence, of the 6,000 physicians in The Permanente Medical Group in Kaiser Permanente's Northern California region, only two left the group because they could not adjust to twenty-first-century approaches requiring the use of an EHR. Moreover, the medical group's current ability to attract and retain high-caliber physicians in every specialty can be attributed, among other factors, to the availability of industry-leading technology.

While we are still learning how to use the technology more efficiently and effectively, none of our physicians would go back to a paper medical record and the limitations of the twentieth century.

—Robert Pearl, MD, executive director and CEO, The Permanente Medical Group

Another predictable issue was concern that physicians would be overwhelmed by e-mail messages from patients. Experience has not borne this out for most physicians, with an average number of e-mail responses sent per provider at 52 per month, or 2.6 per work day. But that is an average, and it varies depending on the specialty (primary care physicians receive more e-mails than neurosurgeons) and also by how strongly the physicians have incorporated the online tools as part of their care routine. Many doctors will see a patient in the clinic, order a test, and suggest that the patient check the result on My Health Manager the next day, or that evening. They may also suggest that the patient send a follow-up e-mail contact in a week or two to report on their progress. These physicians may have a higher volume, but most of them would not go back to the days of playing phone tag with their patients and having to paraphrase the conversation for the medical record. KP HealthConnect automatically saves every single e-mail message sent and received as part of the EHR.

Future Challenges

Currently, My Health Manager on kp.org gives members access to their health data, online programs to improve their health, transactional functionality regarding membership, benefits, and payments, and extensive general health information. The next phase will involve being able to provide appropriate data, programs, and specific health information based on the patient's unique, personal needs and preferences. For example, a patient with a thyroid problem could have features related to their condition brought up automatically when they log on to the site, saving them from having to search the site and displaying information they might not have known to look for. This will require a careful balance between personalizing the site and becoming overly intrusive. In general, though, members say they are eager to see their data transformed into information that is uniquely relevant to their personal situations and that helps them understand what actions they can take to improve their health.

Already, the kp.org site is being redesigned to emphasize the connection between types of data, such as diagnostic, medication, or patient encounter data, and to enhance the ability for members to act on their data to manage their health more collaboratively. This will involve the development of tools that enable patients to incorporate their own data into their PHR, which may or may not be shared with their physician. We believe that combining this capability with mobile devices such as PDAs and cell phones will give patients the ability to track and manage their conditions with tools that fit in with the way they work and live.

Lessons Learned

Following are some of the more important lessons Kaiser Permanente has learned with regard to the implementation and management of online access to patients' medical records. While some of these lessons may be unique to large, multiregional organizations and to PHR-type systems that are integrated with the clinical medical record, most should be relevant to any large health system that seeks to empower their members and patients with extensive and actionable online personal health information.

- Obtain executive-level sponsorship and communicate this support with consistent messages about the benefits and accountabilities, at all leadership levels.
- Identify physician champions who are respected by their colleagues and have strong leadership skills to participate in the planning and to communicate with their colleagues.
- Identify which decisions senior leadership should make and which can be made by physicians and front-line staff. Senior leaders should communicate their decisions and the rationale. As much as possible, involve physicians and front-line staff, including nurses, medical assistants, call center agents, receptionists, and other staff, in decision making. Member advisory groups also provide important input.
- Set the expectation of consensus—that decisions will be made that all can live with—to avoid slowdowns in trying to include everyone's ideas. Live by the slogan, "Perfection is the enemy of the good."
- Involve the "naysayers" early on to address their concerns and learn from their input. They usually have a good reason for saying nay.
- Include representatives from the legal and compliance staffs, and from organized labor, very early in the planning.
- Develop one set of tools that can be adapted to different facets of the organization. Tools can include sample project plans, deployment planning checklists, sample presentations for decisions, presentations to communicate about the project, sample newsletter articles, frequently asked questions to staff, and/or sample marketing materials for the patients.

- Don't start marketing until the system go-live is successful. Even though it looks like everything is working during testing, there can be surprises once something goes live. Marketing a feature to patients as "coming soon" raises expectations that may not be met.
- Promote the online record access using as many different modes as possible. Personal messages from physicians and nurses are most effective.

CHAPTER NINE

IMPROVING PATIENT SAFETY

By Douglas Bonacum

Chapter Summary

A decade after the IOM's alarming report on the risks and dangers of medical care in America, the issue of patient safety remains at the top of the agenda of quality improvement. Part One of this chapter explores the reasons that medical care has traditionally been a hazardous enterprise, and how the development and implementation of electronic health records and decision-support tools can significantly improve patient safety, as they have with the use of KP HealthConnect. Part Two presents four case studies of patient safety-related quality improvement projects that leverage the capabilities of KP HealthConnect.

Part One: Introduction

Every day, thousands of patients are needlessly harmed in the U.S. health care system, and hundreds lose their lives. The statistics are alarming, but even more so are the individual stories of real human beings—patients, doctors, nurses, family members, and others—who have suffered as a result of the level of risk and danger in medical care that for too long has been accepted as the norm. A revealing sampling

Douglas Bonacum, MBA, is vice president for Safety Management at Kaiser Permanente.

of these stories can be viewed and heard on Health Care for All's Website at www.
hcfama.org/quality/stories.

The dimensions of the failure to provide safe medical care first burst into public
awareness with the publication of the Institute of Medicine's seminal report on patient
safety, *To Err Is Human* (Institute of Medicine, 2000), which reported that between
44,000 and 98,000 patients went into U.S. hospitals each year and didn't come out
alive, though not because of what sent them to the hospital. They died from medical
error. This "shot heard around the world" was initially met with some skepticism, but
is now widely recognized and accepted. To put these numbers in some additional
perspective, every day and a half, a fully loaded Boeing 747 airplane would have to
fall from the sky before airline passenger loss of life would surpass hospital patient loss
of life due to medical error. Since then, we have learned the following:

- Nearly two million patients annually get an infection while being treated for another illness or injury, and nearly $5 billion are added to U.S. health costs every
  year as a result of infections that patients acquire while they are hospitalized for
  other health problems (Wenzel, 2001).
- Medication-related errors are estimated to account for about 7,000 deaths each
  year and increase a seven-hundred-bed hospital's annual operating cost by more
  than $3 million annually (Bates and others, 1997).
- According to the Centers for Medicare and Medicaid Services, approximately 1.24
  million patient safety incidents occurred to hospitalized Medicare patients over the
  years 2002–2004. These patient safety incidents were associated with $9.3 billion
  in excess costs and more than 250,000 deaths (Seniorjournal, 2006). As with the
  other statistics provided in this section, this data is specific to what is occurring in
  hospitals with most care provided in the ambulatory arena, for which there have
  been few notable studies of the impact of medical error.

Have things improved since the IOM's *To Err Is Human* report a decade ago? Not
according to numerous recent reports (National Priorities Partnership, 2008; Leapfrog
Group, 2009; Jewell and McGiffert, 2009), all of which acknowledge that while spo-
radic examples of impressive improvements have been achieved in the past decade,
the routine use of evidence-based practices that can improve safety has not been
widespread, and overall progress has been far too slow. How is this possible? Why is
health care so dangerous? The first thing we must appreciate is how complex the
practice of medicine has become. Even with all the medical research that has been
done over the past century, there is not widespread agreement on what constitutes
best practice; diagnosis and treatment are often performed under some degree of
uncertainty; and medication monitoring, particularly in the outpatient setting, is challenging. For a front-line practitioner, there are always new medications, new technologies, new procedures, and new research findings to assimilate. Patients' needs are

becoming increasingly complex, with multiple chronic conditions, and the diversity of the workforce grows at an increasing rate. In addition, there are basic "human factors" that increase our propensity to err, such as fatigue, interruptions and distractions, multitasking, and stress, to name just a few. When an error does occur, the culture of health care is such that individuals are often blamed and shamed while the overall safety and reliability of the underlying system remains the same.

To improve the safety and reliability of care, we must recognize that our historic approach to addressing medical error has been largely ineffective. Thus, concluding that our adverse outcomes are caused by "human errors" committed by a single or a few individuals has done little to improve performance, nor have pursuing risk reduction strategies of didactic education, modifications to policy, and discipline helped. However, by viewing human error as a consequence rather than a cause, laying origins of error not so much in the frailty of human nature as in "upstream" systemic factors, we can implement strategies that more effectively minimize the risk of recurrence by all care givers. Taking a systems-level approach to human error helps an organization improve safety and reliability on the basis of the premise that while we cannot change the human condition, we *can* change the conditions under which humans work. Health information technology systems such as Kaiser Permanente HealthConnect are critical to such a systems-level strategy.

Minimizing Unnecessary Variation

Information technology has the potential to reduce preventable harm or injuries to patients, improve the reliable delivery of evidence-based care, and assist clinicians with complex judgment through the timely provision of information and decision support. While much of this chapter focuses on reducing the risk of preventable harm to patients from the care that is intended to help them, the opportunity to improve the reliability of care—that is, to close the gap between what we know and what we do in health care—is enormous, and so is the opportunity to make better clinical decisions.

A recent, eye-opening Rand Corporation report indicated that adults in the United States received only 55 percent of the care indicated by the best available evidence. The study concluded, "A key component of any solution is the routine availability of information on performance at all levels. Making such information available will require a major overhaul of our current health information systems, with a focus on automating the entry and retrieval of key data" (McGlynn and others, 2003, p. 348).

KP HealthConnect not only automates the entry and retrieval of data, it helps standardize medical practice, where appropriate, to minimize unwarranted variation through the design, implementation, and maintenance of SmartTools, such as shared Order Sets. A KP HealthConnect Order Set for general surgery, for example, includes patient code status (what a patient wants done if they stop breathing or their heart stops beating), specific instructions for nursing and dietary concerns, medications for pain and infection prevention, orders to minimize potentially deadly blood clots, and desired labs as applicable. As new evidence emerges, the Order Sets can be efficiently updated and all surgeons can make clinical decisions guided by the best available research, right at their fingertips. Such tools allow physicians to focus on customizing care to the particular patient's condition rather than on remembering routine recommendations.

Moving beyond issues of reliability, information technology is becoming more and more important to support clinical decision making, both across the continuum of care and over a patient's lifetime. With a paper chart, practitioners (when they can locate the chart) have what is called "encounter-level data"—that is, data that is true as of a given event. While it can be viewed over time, it represents information as of a *moment* in time, such as orders placed in a particular visit, documentation of symptoms or physical findings on a particular visit, and assessment of a patient in a visit with recommendations based on that assessment.

An electronic health record (EHR), however, can provide what is called "patient-level data" that is true for a patient over time, not just on a given day or linked to a particular encounter. Much like demographic information, it may be verified at each encounter, but it is not redocumented at each encounter unless it has changed. Examples include allergies, medications, the problem list, medical and surgical history, and social history.

Having patient-level data is not only more efficient (that is, practitioners don't have to individually and repetitively record the same information again and again in different pages of a medical ledger), it is more effective. Care givers can now *share* a database that centers on the patient. From a patient safety perspective, the first improvement is simply the ability to access meaningful data in the moment that may have been generated long ago. More important, computerized clinical decision support based on patient-level data can improve practitioner decision making by matching an individual patient's characteristics in the computerized knowledge base with powerful software algorithms that deliver information and recommendations to the clinician almost instantaneously. Physicians still have the opportunity to practice the art of medicine, but they are now guided by science and technology.

Refocusing on Systems Versus Individuals

Returning to the goal of reducing preventable harm or injuries to patients, we have found the following framework helpful: much of the preventable harm to patients receiving health care today appears to be caused by the very practitioners who are trying to help them. That said, whether it be a simple human error or an inadvertent procedural violation, we will not achieve break-through levels of safety and reliability by focusing on individuals in the aftermath of adverse outcomes, by blaming them for forgetfulness, inattention, or even ignorance of the latest science. A better approach to human fallibility is to focus more on the conditions under which individuals and teams work. Here, workflow patterns and systemic defenses are designed to avert errors, the conditions that lend themselves to violations are minimized, and mechanisms are put in place to mitigate harm when mistakes nevertheless occur.

Borrowing from industrial safety science and a concept known as the "hierarchy of controls," Kaiser Permanente developed a model to help assess the likelihood of reducing risk and improving reliability through systemic changes, as shown in Figure 9.1. The theory behind this model is that there is a logical order of effectiveness that a system designer or process owner can use to evaluate the potential efficacy of a host of "controls." Controls can be thought of as mechanisms to help ensure that a simplified, standardized process functions over time as designed. For example, within KP HealthConnect, a safety alert generated by a medication order for a particularly hazardous drug may be more effective in reducing harm than a policy regarding prescription practices. Building on that example, removal of the particularly harmful medication from the prescriber's drug

FIGURE 9.1. A HIERARCHY OF CONTROLS FOR REDUCING RISK.

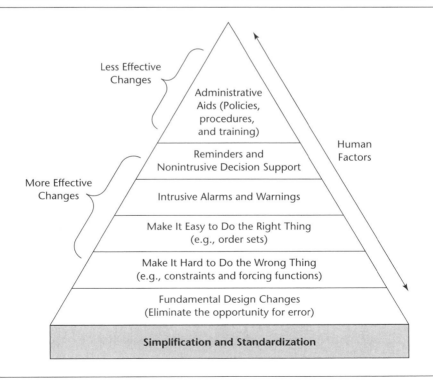

formulary—the list of drugs at his disposal—and from local storage bins (fundamental design changes), where feasible, may be even more effective than the alert.

Approach and Principles

The primary objective of a safe system design is to make it difficult for individuals to err, to address errors when they nonetheless occur, and to monitor performance over time. With an eye toward that objective, the strategy we use at Kaiser Permanente to improve patient safety through KP HealthConnect is guided by the following approach:

- Identify areas of risk to patient safety;
- Evaluate the likelihood of reducing risk and/or improving reliability through KP HealthConnect; and
- Assess other factors, such as impact on clinical workflow, ease of use, and patient preferences, to further help prioritize improvement opportunities.

Assessing factors such as impact on clinical workflow, ease of use, and patient preferences is largely done by operations managers within the organization. Clinical quality, patient safety, and clinical risk management leaders play an extensive role in partnering with operations to identify areas of risk and evaluate the likelihood of improved performance through KP HealthConnect.

Areas of risk to patient safety are primarily identified through analysis of our own internally reported events; benchmarking with other industry leaders and organizations, such as the IHI; and review of the literature. Key opportunities we have identified include medication safety, improving the timeliness and reliability of diagnosis, and patient engagement to improve patient safety. When considering the likelihood of improving performance in these areas with the aid of technology, we are guided by the hierarchy of controls coupled with the following "human factors" design principles:

- *Minimize variation in practice*—Simplifying and standardizing the structure of tasks to help minimize the pressure on vulnerable cognitive processes such as working memory;
- *Reduce reliance on memory*—Avoiding reliance on memory while increasing vigilance to minimize the risk of slips and lapses using a wide variety of tools available in KP HealthConnect, including standard Order Sets, reminders, and in-basket reports;
- *Improve access to information*—Improving clinical decision making and reducing reliance on memory by providing easy online access to a wide range of electronic reference materials on drugs and diseases at the point of care, as well as patient-level data across time and space;

- *Flag harm*—Using visual controls in the EHR to help focus attention, such as flagging abnormal lab or test results and providing out-of-range indicators;
- *Use constraints and "force functions"*—Providing intelligent decision support to mitigate uncertainties and deploying redundant alerts, including medication dosing alerts, drug formulary checks, or drug-drug interaction alerts, where appropriate, to "force" the capture and mitigation of an error before it has the chance to do harm;
- *Facilitate follow-up*—Examples include "tickler," or reminder, messages that providers can send themselves regarding a specific item they want to check on in the future, flagging tests ordered but not completed, and requiring a practitioner to remotely cover a vacationing practitioner's in-basket so that key lab and test results are not delayed or lost to follow-up; and
- *Engage the patient as partner in safety*—Connecting patients to their health care team and personal health information system via KP HealthConnect's Web-based member portal, which allows them to view most test results, send secure messages to their doctor, check their past visit information, and access their post-visit patient instructions, provides additional checks on the care process.

The following section describes some specific patient safety-related applications that have emerged from these overall approaches and principles.

Practical Applications

By benchmarking with other industry leaders who had implemented an electronic health record, we recognized before deploying KP HealthConnect that there would be immediate patient safety benefits from the mere implementation of our EHR. The patient safety "glass," if you will, comes partially filled, through mechanisms described in Figure 9.2.

Following the system's go-live and stabilization phase, we activated the existing functionality for enhanced patient safety, advised by the approach and guiding principles described in the previous section. Examples of such features are depicted in Figure 9.3.

As we gained increased comfort with KP HealthConnect and better understood its potential to transform the way that health care is delivered, we looked for ways to accelerate patient safety performance by

- Streamlining workflow;
- Preventing, catching, and correcting errors;
- Offering higher level decision-support; and
- Monitoring performance.

These approaches are illustrated in Figure 9.4.

FIGURE 9.2. IMMEDIATE SAFETY BENEFITS OF THE EHR.

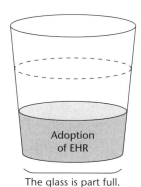

The glass is part full.

Examples of Safety Benefits

• Patient-level data

• Legibility: readable and organized patient information

• Ubiquitous access to patient's medical record 24/7

• Longitudinal medical problem list that can be maintained and transitioned across settings

• Longitudinal record of all historical and current medications, immunizations, and lab results

FIGURE 9.3. LEVERAGING EXISTING FUNCTIONALITY AND FEATURES.

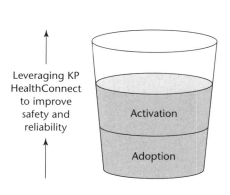

Leveraging KP HealthConnect to improve safety and reliability

Examples

• Drug–drug interaction alerts

• Health maintenance reminders

• Best practice alerts

• Order sets configured to standardize practice based on evidence base

• Dose restrictions for specific drugs

• After visit summary reports for patient/family

• KP HealthConnect Online linking patients to their health care team and personal health system

FIGURE 9.4. ACCELERATING PATIENT SAFETY PERFORMANCE.

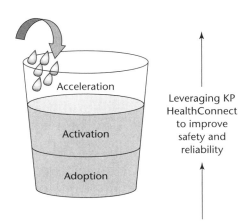

- Closing the loop on lab and test results

- Enhancing computerized physician order entry

- Barcoding

- Refining decision support

- Creating surveillance systems for drug use

- Exploring new ways to detect harm

Acceleration

Activation

Adoption

Leveraging KP HealthConnect to improve safety and reliability

Specific Patient Safety Initiatives

A closer look at several of the initiatives noted in Figures 9.3 and 9.4 follows as well as a number of other related improvements that further highlight the practical applications and innovative enhancements that have been made to KP HealthConnect. Several of these initiatives are more explicitly described in the case studies at the end of this chapter.

Closing the Loop on Lab and Test Results

Health care organizations have struggled for years to implement a "safety net" to close the loop on delays and failures throughout the life cycle of a clinical order. Historically, many organizations have used a combination of paper-based and human communication systems as a way to transmit orders and receive order results. These systems are highly susceptible to human errors (for example, paper results lost or mishandled, breakdown in communication between clinicians and/or to patients) and do not ensure adequate outreach to members due for preventive measures (for example, breast cancer screening). The physician challenges include

- Volume of data to be reviewed by each physician is large (one study indicates it could be as high as more than eight hundred results per week) (Gandhi, 2005);
- Availability of test results range from less than an hour to weeks after the tests are ordered;
- Ability to contact patients to follow up on results can be difficult;
- Paper-based test reporting systems are subject to delivery delays and misfiling; and
- Specialists in testing areas may not have adequate clinical information about why the test was ordered and do not have clear criteria for which results require urgent notification.

Multiple studies and publications have documented the delays and failures that can occur in the life cycle of an outpatient diagnostic or laboratory order. One study of patients in five countries found that 8 percent to 20 percent of adults who were treated as outpatients did not receive their test results, and 9 percent to 15 percent received incorrect results or delayed notification of abnormal results (Schoen and others, 2004). Another indicated that the failure to get test results into the right hands with the right follow-up was a significant source of malpractice (Gandhi and others, 2006). In short, "closing the loop" is a top patient safety priority for all health care organizations, with the key opportunities including an order being transmitted but not performed, an order being performed but the result not being reviewed, or the result being reviewed but not acted upon.

Kaiser Permanente is testing several strategies to improve the reliability of "closing the loop." These include

- Utilizing the "Overdue Results Notification" functionality in KP HealthConnect, which sends in-basket messages to the provider for ordered tests and procedures that are not completed within a specified time period. From the in-basket, staff or physicians can then write letters to patients asking them to come in for their missed tests, a process facilitated by the ability to select a blank letter template that can be quickly customized for the patient using a KP HealthConnect tool called "SmartText."
- Using several available reports to monitor the overall performance of the system. These include a monthly "Abnormal Lab Results" monitoring report, as shown in Figure 9.5, which shows the number of unread abnormal lab results messages more than fourteen days old in the in-basket, and an "In-Basket Management Report" that shows the age and volume of messages in the in-basket. Not only can these reports provide summary statistics, they can be accompanied by more detailed lists by department or provider for use in performance improvement activities. As an example, the Abnormal Lab Results report includes a list of locations and

FIGURE 9.5. IN-BASKET VIEW—ABNORMAL RESULT.

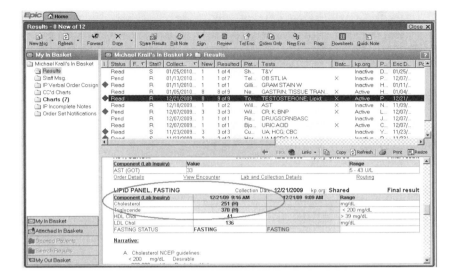

Configuring the provider's in-basket view to demonstrate abnormal results in a way that facilitates follow-up.

providers with unread abnormal lab result messages in their in-basket that are reviewed by Physician Directors and/or Team Leaders for monitoring and follow-up, as indicated. Such follow-up includes

- Improved workflows for closing the in-baskets of providers who have transferred locations or left Kaiser Permanente;
- Development of departmental coverage agreements to cover providers who are out of the office for extended periods of time; and
- Provision of general and individualized training for improved in-basket management.

Computerized Physician Order Entry (CPOE)

Studies showing improved patient safety from EHR use in hospital and ambulatory care largely focus on alerts, reminders, and other components of CPOE (Bates and others, 1999). These are not necessarily "off the shelf" features and typically need to be developed or refined by an organization to maximize effectiveness. CPOE makes important safety information available to the physician and/or pharmacist before a medication is dispensed. An example might be a warning about potential interactions with a patient's other drugs for a new drug the physician orders. (See the sidebar "Managing Medication-Related Alerts" near the end of this chapter.) Where appropriate, best-practice alerts can be linked to the safety alert not only to warn prescribers about the potential risk of their decision but also to offer alternative medications.

For example, metformin is a drug generally used to control blood sugar levels in people with Type 1 diabetes. Some patients on this drug were arriving for a CT scan with contrast to provide a greater visual differentiation between normal and abnormal tissue. However, the interaction between the contrast agent and this diabetes medication can contribute to kidney damage. Now, when a provider orders a CT scan with contrast for a diabetic taking metformin, a drug-drug interaction fires what is called a "Best Practice Alert," such as, "SAFETY ALERT: This imaging study is performed with contrast and this patient has Metformin on their medication list. Open SmartSet for instructions and follow-up lab recommendations." The SmartSet template contains the default order, standardized progress note, and patient follow-up instructions per FDA guidelines. In this case, the guidelines noted the following: "(1) stop metformin after the CT scan/Imaging procedure, (2) test creatinine level 48 hours post-scan, and (3) evaluate creatinine level prior to patient restarting medication."

In addition, a default set of patient instructions in the After Visit Summary gives patients written instructions to reinforce their discussion with the practitioner. The After Visit Summary can also be viewed by the patient online from My Health Manager in kp.org at any time. A typical patient instruction, for instance, might read, "You are having a CT scan that requires you STOP taking your DIABETIC MEDICATION METFORMIN AFTER you have your test. You MUST also have a LAB TEST 48 HOURS after your CT scan. Go to any Kaiser Lab and have this test done 48 hours after your CT scan. Please CONTACT YOUR DOCTOR AFTER YOU HAVE YOUR LAB TEST and your doctor will tell you when it is safe to resume taking the Metformin."

Barcoding

What CPOE offers on the "front-end" of the medication management process (that is, prescribing), barcoding offers on the "back-end" (that is, administering). A barcode is an optical machine-readable representation of data, most commonly seen in supermarket checkout systems. Data is encoded on both the medication and the patient (on a wristband), both of which are scanned at the point of care.

While studies conducted in VA hospitals in the early 1990s showed that the use of barcodes reduced medication administration error rates by up to 86 percent (Meadows,

2003), estimates presented at a recent patient safety conference sponsored by the Center for Business Innovation indicate that only 2 percent to 6 percent of hospitals are currently using them to reduce medication administration errors. At Kaiser Permanente, every hospital is implementing barcoding with KP HealthConnect.

Although nurses are still trained and held accountable for the so-called "Five Rights" of medication administration (right patient, right medication, right dose, right route, and right time), barcoding offers an additional set of checks and balances at the point of medication administration. An assessment of early results is impressive. In one of our medical centers, the medication administration error rate has decreased by over 50 percent; in another, the percentage of medication and armband overrides documented in KP HealthConnect dropped from 27 percent to 7 percent; and at a third center, such overrides dropped from 13 percent to 4 percent.

Like any new technological solution, barcoding does not come without a new set of problems. In addition to the challenge of learning a new technology, there are changes in workflow that need to be designed as well. Also, nurses may be confronted with system glitches that can drive the use of workarounds in order to complete their tasks on time. The following account provides further insight into the challenges one of our medical centers faced and what staff and management did together to successfully address them.

Rescuing Patient Safety Issues from the "Black Hole"

In Southern California, Kaiser Permanente's regional and local Quality and Risk Management (QRM) departments track KP HealthConnect-related quality and patient safety issues, including those linked with operations and workflows. Yet, many felt these issues were going into a "black hole"—concerns were being reported, but the perception was that nothing was being done to address them. What was needed was a forum for collaboration between KP HealthConnect experts and staff working in operations to openly discuss these quality/patient safety issues in a blame-free atmosphere. We created such a forum in the KP HealthConnect Quality of Care and Patient Safety Oversight Committee.

KP HealthConnect quality/patient safety issues are received via many venues, including an intranet database, which provides a transparent forum for regional and local issue reporting and resolutions, and related communications. All medical centers have received training in the use of this venue.

Reported issues are reviewed at least monthly with the respective KP HealthConnect application leads, and those with region-wide impact are discussed during the oversight committee meeting. Committee members and ad hoc subject matter experts clarify whether issues are user issues, workflow issues, and/or KP HealthConnect application issues and develop solutions that may include workflow redesign, end-user training, or application enhancements. In addition, committee members coordinate various patient safety workgroups in support of major regional and national initiatives that have linkages between operations and KP HealthConnect.

In order to address the perception of the "black hole," an executive summary of the committee's work is distributed widely to regional and local quality and risk management leaders and key stakeholders, and committee members are encouraged to share them with the peer groups they represent.

For the committee to be successful, a collaborative spirit and an emphasis on just culture must be developed. It is imperative that operations, EHR application leads, and ad hoc experts analyze both technical and human factor issues and work collaboratively to identify and disseminate solutions.

—By Pamela Wald, MD, assistant area medical director, and Betsey Haren,
director of Clinical Information and Performance Evaluation,
Kaiser Permanente-Southern California

Improving the Reliability of Care

While the evidence for many practices in medicine is not firm, developing a consistent baseline of care when there is sufficient evidence promotes learning and performance improvement. By establishing shared protocols for care at Kaiser Permanente, we can make good judgments using the evidence we have, implement those choices together, measure the results, and improve practice over time. One such example of this approach is the development and use of shared Order Sets within KP HealthConnect.

Reducing Hospital-Associated Pneumonia.

All of our medical centers have an aim to eliminate ventilator-associated pneumonia, or VAP. Pneumonia accounts for approximately 15 percent of all hospital-associated infections and 27 percent and 24 percent of all infections acquired in the medical intensive-care unit (ICU) and coronary care unit (CCU), respectively. It has been the second most common hospital-associated infection after that of the urinary tract. The primary risk factor for the development of hospital-associated bacterial pneumonia is mechanical ventilation, with its requisite endotracheal intubation (Centers for Disease Control and Prevention, 2005). Despite the frequency of occurrence, VAPs are considered preventable. The Institute for Healthcare Improvement (IHI) has provided information on the prevention of VAP in the form of scientifically grounded steps referred to as care bundles, which have been shown to reduce VAP rates (Institute for Healthcare Improvement, n.d.).

In 2005, Kaiser Permanente's Baldwin Park Medical Center in Los Angeles set a goal of zero incidences of VAP, established in concert with the IHI's "Saving 100,000 Lives Campaign." The strategy was to establish paper-based protocols that included IHI's ventilator bundle (a set of five practices that when done together have been shown to improve safety), hand washing, and oral hygiene. Daily multidisciplinary rounds were also established, led by an ICU physician and attended by all appropriate staff, including RNs and pharmacists. The average incident rate in 2005 was 3.0 per one thousand patient days. In October 2006, with KP HealthConnect implementation, the same protocols were embedded into KP HealthConnect ICU Order Sets relating to admissions, invasive ventilation, and sedation. As a result of having these protocols embedded in the EHR, the average incident rate dropped 60 percent in the first year of implementation in 2007. Since then, the cumulative rate is 1.6 per thousand days, representing a sustained reduction of 36 percent below the pre-intervention rate of 2.5.

We continue to look for new ways to leverage KP HealthConnect to improve patient safety and reliability. We do this also with awareness that some of our decisions may have inadvertently created risk. The next section describes several mechanisms we have in place to address this issue.

Managing Unforeseen Risks

Kaiser Permanente went into the implementation of KP HealthConnect recognizing that with every new solution comes a new set of challenges. While KP HealthConnect had the potential to help address a number of complex challenges, a number of articles in the literature suggested the jury was still out regarding proven outcomes (for example, Wears and Berg, 2005). In addition, some of the studies we reviewed indicated that risk could actually be increased through the adoption of technology, not decreased. For example, researchers conducting separate studies in the United States, the Netherlands, and Australia, using similar qualitative methods to investigate implementing patient care IT systems, encountered many instances in which system applications seemed to foster errors rather than reduce their likelihood. The errors appeared to fall into two main categories: those in the process of entering and retrieving information and those in the communication and coordination process that the clinical information system is supposed to support (Ash, Berg, and Coiera, 2004).

Our approach to managing unforeseen risk has been multidimensional, including the establishment of a national technology remediation process and the development of regional mechanisms to assess, prioritize, and track through resolution quality of care and patient safety issues that are identified and can be managed at the local level (see sidebar earlier in this chapter).

A National Help Desk and remediation process called PART has been established to address issues that cannot be managed at the local level, such as broader system issues that may lead to inaccurate, misleading, or incomplete patient care information. The acronym PART stands for the main steps of the process:

- *Preparation*—clarifies the incident report, rules out user error, and determines if the incident is to be reported as potential risk to patient safety;
- *Assessment*—determines urgency on the basis of severity, scope, and likelihood of occurrence, what immediate action is needed, and which regions are impacted;
- *Remediation*—refines the analysis of impact and develops a plan of action addressing immediate mitigation and longer-term resolution, and determines remediation; and
- *Track*—tracks the incident to completion and validates successful remediation.

PART helps determine the extent of the potential patient safety issue, facilitate the development of an action plan, and communicate widely. The process engages appropriate groups when formulating solutions and ensures that the individuals who need to know about the issue hear about it in a timely manner. Incidents identified as potential patient safety issues are addressed and resolved within two to twenty-four hours. The national KP HealthConnect team, made up of representatives from regions by an incident, appropriate subject matter experts, and our partners from Epic, are paged to a bridge call and convene immediately to take action to mitigate the problem and put into place any workarounds. Since 2005, there have been more than six hundred issues identified and remedied.

Part Two: Select Patient Safety Initiatives with KP HealthConnect

Following are detailed descriptions of four important patient safety initiatives involving the use of KP HealthConnect, contributed by clinicians and other patient safety experts involved in their development.

Automated Harm Detection

Detecting harm that occurs in health care delivery systems has traditionally relied on voluntary reporting or tracking of errors, and the level of reporting has been generally unsatisfactory. A relatively new approach using "trigger tools" is a more reliable way to identify adverse events and quantify the risk, degree, and severity of harm, a way that allows hospitals to select and test interventions to prevent harm (Classen and others, 2008).

Triggers are defined as signals or "red flags" found within a medical record that may indicate harm experienced by the patient and the need for further investigation to determine the presence or absence of an adverse event. The IHI has led the development of trigger tools and related methodology for both specific and global triggers. Specific trigger tools look at individual care delivery activities, such as medication or surgery, while the Global Trigger Tool looks at the overall health care delivery system. Although the Global Trigger Tool was originally designed to detect adverse events and not near misses, organizations can use positive triggers without associated harm as a measure of risk. The federal Agency for Healthcare Research and Quality has recommended the IHI Global Trigger Tool as the preferred means of measuring harm in health care delivery systems.

KP HealthConnect allows Kaiser Permanente to augment the typically manually intensive IHI methodology in two important and innovative ways: it can search the medical records of *all* hospitalized patients instead of a random sample, and it can provide information in near real time. As of 2009, this automated surveillance approach was being piloted at our Antioch Medical Center in the Northern California region. The center's quality/safety/risk management department generates a daily report that identifies all positive triggers associated with the medical record of any patient currently in the hospital, and safety/quality issues are referred to treating physicians as needed. On the basis of the identification of positive triggers, there have been several instances when the quality department has been able to proactively alert a patient's health care team to minimize or even prevent an adverse event. The ability to accomplish this in near real time is only possible with the use of an electronic record.

The ability to use KP HealthConnect to perform automated trigger surveillance is a powerful means of detecting and decreasing harm to patients, but it is not without its limitations. Challenges to the automated process include variable data quality, multiple data sources, variation in the operational definition of data elements, and capacity demands—both human and technological. With a clear understanding of the relationship between operational workflows and database capabilities, and ongoing evaluation of the use and value of automated surveillance reports, hospitals can use the EHRs to enhance the identification, prevention, and mitigation of harm and proactively identify performance improvement opportunities.

—Dot Snow, MPH, national lead for KP HealthConnect and Patient Safety, National Patient Safety

The Emergency Medical Risk Initiative

Despite several ongoing, targeted risk reduction initiatives, the frequency of medical malpractice claims made against Kaiser Permanente has remained relatively flat for the past few years, with slight severity increases year over year. Close to half of these claims result from diagnosis-related issues. An exhaustive Kaiser Permanente study of the causes of these adverse events revealed opportunities for systematic improvements in every stage of the diagnostic process. The events, however, were not grouped into a particular setting or medical specialty. The only isolated setting for which we could identify a clear grouping was the emergency department (ED), which was the setting for about 11 percent of all diagnosis-related claims. We also determined that the course of treatment for about 40 percent of all diagnosis-related cases included an encounter with an ED.

The initial search for a targeted education intervention for the ED led to a comprehensive system for risk reduction by the Sullivan Group. The system focuses on the diagnostic process to help eliminate a failure or delay in diagnosis and includes clinical content for diagnostic decision support, clinical risk reduction education, and regular feedback to clinicians regarding their documentation performance. The decision support, in the form of risk prompts that serve as physician reminders, prevents cognitive traps and leads to more complete documentation in the medical record.

A test of this system, known as the Emergency Medicine Risk Initiative (EMRI), was commissioned in 2005 to assess the applicability of the EMRI program to Kaiser Permanente. The goals were to

- Demonstrate that a prompted medical record will improve the quality of physician documentation as measured by the EMRI audit;
- Test a systematic program of continuous improvement for management of emergency medicine risk that includes education, real-time bedside tools, and a performance assessment; and
- Assess the feasibility of incorporation of the decision support, audit, and reporting functionality into KP HealthConnect.

Five Kaiser Permanente EDs piloted the program using a manual version of the decision support/prompting documentation tool. This demonstration included a pre- and post-audit of a sample of records to determine compliance with specified risk factor documentation. In addition, the educational component was evaluated.

The manual tool resulted in improved scores on the clinical documentation audit and increased compliance in gathering information and acting on key indicators of patient risk. For maximum adoption and benefit, the pilot experience confirmed the need to incorporate the decision-support elements into the flow of the EHR.

A survey of pilot site physicians about their experience with the system found that 41 percent of respondents were using prompts and found them helpful; 88 percent had taken online education and found it helpful; and medical record audit feedback helped improve documentation and diagnosis. On the basis of the pilots, it was decided that the chart template containing the decision-support elements and the audit and monitoring program would be incorporated in the KP HealthConnect collaborative build for all Kaiser Permanente EDs.

—Mark Littlewood , director, Risk Management and Patient Safety,
The Permanente Federation

Clinical Decision Support: Making the Right Thing Easy to Do

Clinical decision support at the point of care is one of the principal opportunities for patient safety and quality improvement offered by EHRs such as KP HealthConnect. The U.S. Office of the National Coordinator of Health Information Technology, among others, has recognized decision support as fundamental to achieving significant benefit and "meaningful use" of EHR systems. Delivering effective decision support, however, poses many challenges, including

- Capturing discrete ("coded") data required by the system to make accurate inferences;
- Choosing the interaction model (optional versus automatic) and display mode (intrusive versus non-intrusive) appropriate to the situation;
- Considering workflow and human factors, including limitations of human attention and cognition;
- General clinical information overload and the real and perceived impact of decision support leading to "alert fatigue;" and
- Barriers to adoption and use of clinical content generally and decision support in particular.

Given these considerations, useful decision support in a particular domain and circumstance might be a well-designed flow sheet or report, perhaps with a particular cell or value highlighted to draw the user's attention. In other cases, available access to advisories, results of prioritization or predictive modeling, or context-specific knowledge resources might be optimal. Finally, certain situations warrant intrusive alerting with optional or required responses (so called "forcing functions"). In all cases, and particularly as intrusiveness (and thus workflow interruption) increases, effective decision support must be accurate, important, relevant, and actionable.

KP HealthConnect contains many examples of effective clinical decision support. We learned early on that achieving benefit involves more than simply building excellent tools. Reports by region and by department demonstrated wide variation in use, with those departments that had active and engaged KP HealthConnect leaders and local champions far exceeding the use of safety-related decision support tools compared to those that did not. All Kaiser Permanente regions have built clinical evidence and guidance into ordering and charting templates, such as "SmartSets" and "Order Sets." All regions have also implemented both nonintrusive and intrusive alerts and advisories.

The Northwest region in 2009, for example, had more than seventy custom medication safety alerts, divided about equally into drug-drug interactions, drug-condition appropriateness, prescribing in the elderly, and renal dosing issues. In addition, there were more than fifty other safety-related advisories, mostly focused on recognizing high-risk diagnoses in the ED. Following implementation of alerts for high-risk drugs in the elderly, these prescriptions showed a sustained improvement of about 22 percent compared to baseline. A similar alert, triggered when the anti-nausea medication promethazine was prescribed in children under the age of two years, reduced this hazardous event to essentially zero. In addition to warning against risk, these alerts suggest and facilitate preferred prescriptions or actions, thus going beyond "making it hard to err" to "making it easy to do the right thing," which un-questionably constitutes meaningful use.

—Michael Krall, MD , Kaiser Permanente-Northwest
Clinical Content and Decision Support Lead

Managing Medication-Related Alerts

The integration of real-time, in-process decision support tools within EHRs holds great promise for improving quality and patient safety by intercepting potentially problem-atic orders before they are carried out. Frequently cited examples of these tools are those related to drug-drug, drug-food, drug-disease, minimum/maximum doses, and drug "allergy" screening. CPOE systems are typically designed to pop up alert mes-sages when a medication order is matched with a potential problem in the systems' databases. Most CPOE systems utilize clinical content databases for medications from commercial providers (for example, First DataBank® or MediSpan®).

The advantage, both clinically and operationally, is that the prescriber can modify offending medication orders in real-time, before the medication order is passed to the patient and/or the pharmacy. Historically, drug-related problems were initially screened and identified downstream from initiation of the order, at the pharmacy processing the prescription. The pharmacist would then need to put the patient on hold while the prescriber was contacted to resolve the medication-related alert that fired within the pharmacy system.

Kaiser Permanente's expectations and assumptions when we began work with our vendors to design and implement a CPOE system (both for inpatients and outpa-tients) was that we would get the following medication-related alerts, and that these alerts would be appropriately targeted to situations of true clinical validity:

- Drug allergy checking;
- Basic dosing guidance (dose range checking);
- Formulary decision support;
- Duplicate therapy checking; and
- Drug-drug interaction (DDI) checking.

As we gained experience with the system, it was clear that the acceptance rate for the vast majority of the drug-related alerts was unacceptably low (less than 10 percent), and complaints from prescribers about "irrelevant alerts" and "too many alerts" rose exponentially. We realized that to optimize the utility of decision-support alerts, we would need to work very closely with the system vendor(s) to ensure that the CPOE software appropriately utilizes the clinical content database. We also needed to obtain data necessary to evaluate the appropriateness of DDI alerts and to devise a process to do that. And finally, we needed a clinically and operationally credible process for the ongoing evaluation of alert data to take informed action to improve selectivity, sensitivity, and specificity of alerts to avoid "alert fatigue."

Kaiser Permanente's medication alert management process now incorporates at least the following activities:

- Actual case experience within Kaiser Permanente that involved significant adverse events;
- Comprehensive review of recent look-back data regarding actual alert rates and acceptance rates; and
- Compelling evidence from internal Kaiser Permanente clinicians and/or external expert sources that our DDI severity levels need modification.

As a result of these early challenges and our ongoing determination to improve the clinical validity of decision-support alerts, we now have moved from a less than 10 percent acceptance rate for severe DDI prescriber alerts to a current 2009 rate of more than 30 percent, which exceeds what is most frequently cited in the literature. We will continue our dogged determination to improve the sensitivity, selectivity, and specificity of all medication-related alerts, with a goal that all drug-related alerts are accepted at least 50 percent of the time.

—Carey Cotterell, RPh, pharmacy quality and patient safety leader,
Kaiser Permanente-Southern California

Conclusion

Every day, throughout the entire health care enterprise, the best, the brightest, and the most committed make mistakes. Diagnoses are missed, orders are misunderstood, and medications are administered incorrectly. Yet exhorting providers to try harder, to slow down, or to be more vigilant isn't working.

Information technology has the potential to reduce preventable harm or injuries to patients, improve the reliable delivery of evidence-based care, and assist clinicians with complex judgment through the provision of information and decision support. Leveraging human factor principles that have proven to be successful in other high-risk industries (for example, commercial aviation, nuclear power generation, high-speed rail transportation, chemical manufacturing), a fully accessible and integrated electronic health record system, with instant access to up-to-date medical information, can help right many of the wrongs that patients experience today.

Taking a systems-level approach to human error does not eliminate harm, but it can dramatically help an organization address safety and reliability issues that have otherwise remained beyond our ability to affect.

CHAPTER TEN

SUPERCHARGING RESEARCH THROUGH KP HEALTHCONNECT

By Mary L. Durham, PhD

Chapter Summary

This chapter examines the many ways in which the electronic health record (EHR) and the vast amount of clinical data it provides have benefited clinical research at Kaiser Permanente and other research institutions. Using summaries of recent Kaiser Permanente-sponsored research studies, the author discusses how KP HealthConnect and earlier EHRs have been used to enable population-based research that is improving patient safety, chronic care management, and quality measurement and outcomes—research that was previously impractical due to lack of data or rapid analytic processing power. The author also discusses the use of the EHR to enable new prospective studies of vaccine safety and real-time surveillance, comparative effectiveness, and personalized medicine based on vast genetic and genomic databases, all of which have important implications for improved public health. The chapter concludes with a review of three recent research studies based on data derived from KP HealthConnect.

Mary L. Durham is director of Kaiser Permanente's Center for Health Research in Portland, Oregon, and vice president of research for Kaiser Foundation Hospitals.

Introduction

Kaiser Permanente has been conducting health care research since 1943, one year after our first hospital opened its doors in Oakland, California. From the beginning, scientific discovery has been essential to the organization's mission. Cofounder Henry Kaiser believed that one of the major goals of the organization was to provide funds for research. Today, Kaiser Permanente has eight research centers across the country that conduct epidemiological studies and health services research. It is one of the largest nongovernmental and nonacademic research programs in the United States.

Kaiser Permanente's research technology has evolved dramatically over the decades—from pulling files and abstracting data by hand, one chart at a time, to Serial Attached SCSI programming that involves instant exchanges of trillions of blocks of electronic medical data between storage devices. One of the enormous milestones in the evolution of Kaiser Permanente's research technology was the decision to implement an EHR, which came about in the 1990s. Not surprisingly, the research community embraced it immediately. In fact, the EHR was the product of a long, slow transition that had begun decades earlier.

Researchers were some of the earliest creators and users of the pre–Kaiser Permanente HealthConnect versions of the EHR. As early as 1966, Kaiser Permanente-Northwest's Center for Health Research (CHR) launched OPUS, a population-based medical record system that continuously updated a random sampling of membership data. The tumor registry, started in the 1960s, went online in 1970, pathology records in 1971, and inpatient medical records in 1978. During the 1980s, CHR had access to databases for cytology, outside claims and referrals, outpatient pharmacy, and radiology.

Also in the 1960s, the Northern California region's Department of Research (DOR) began automating its medical records using punch cards. By 1973, every Kaiser Permanente member in Northern California had a computerized medical record.

The Colorado region's Institute of Health Research in 1991 created a data backbone for research outcomes called Integrated Services Information System that coordinated various datasets, including outpatient, hospital, and emergency room utilization and cost estimates into one relational platform. In the mid-1990s, Colorado collaborated with IBM to develop its pre–KP HealthConnect electronic medical record, called the Clinical Information System, which it used until the region adopted KP HealthConnect in 2005. In the same period, a Permanente physician and IT specialist in the Ohio region developed and deployed an in-house EHR system called MARS, for Medical Automated Record System.

Despite all this activity, before the advent of KP HealthConnect, data remained diffuse, spread out among the organization's operating regions in different formats on various platforms. So when the organization took its first steps toward a unified health information technology in the mid-1990s, the research community was thrilled with the data potential. Rather than our usual surveys or record reviews of populations of interest, we would be able to make ever-improving data queries covering the entire membership, increasing our research capacity exponentially. It would be the beginning of a new era: we really would be able to identify quickly, for example, the number of diabetic women between the ages of forty-five and sixty. In addition, the obvious advantage of having clinical information for our entire membership would give tremendous heft to our research proposals to the National Institutes of Health (NIH).

That promise was finally fulfilled when Kaiser Permanente began the system-wide implementation of KP HealthConnect in 2003. Today we are in a position to take full advantage of the EHR in research.

EHR-Enabled Population Research

A stellar example of EHR-fueled research is a landmark study in gestational diabetes mellitus (GDM) led by endocrinologist and diabetes expert Teresa Hillier, MD, MS, a senior CHR investigator in the Northwest and Hawaii regions. Kaiser Permanente has long screened for and treated GDM, but in 2000, national guidelines for GDM diagnosis changed, lowering the threshold and thus increasing prevalence. Under these expanded criteria, roughly 50 percent more women suddenly "became" GDM patients, falling within the new guidelines, while previously their glucose levels would have been considered within normal range (Ferrara and others, 2002). Therefore, while women with more severe GDM had always been treated, Kaiser Permanente began to treat a new cohort with milder GDM.

Hillier saw this as a unique epidemiological opportunity to study GDM outcomes. She was able to compare milder cases of "untreated" GDM (women whose glucose was considered normal before the new guidelines) with treated GDM (women with the worst, or highest, glucose levels, who had always been treated). By studying the electronic records of these cohorts, Hillier was able to test a hypothesis she had long held: that GDM caused metabolic imprinting in the fetus, manifesting later as an increased risk of childhood obesity.

In one of our most influential research studies of 2007, Hillier and her colleagues found that five to seven years after delivery, the children of "untreated" GDM mothers were nearly twice as likely to be overweight (Hillier and others, 2007). Researchers also found that the increased risk of childhood obesity disappeared if the mother's GDM had been treated—even among severe cases. As a result of this study, the Northwest region revised its protocols for screening and treating pregnant women at risk for GDM. This research will improve the health of thousands of people in two generations and, because obesity has lifelong implications, this discovery has lasting effects for many more years to come. Hillier is now advancing her GDM research in a new prospective study for which she is working to diagnose and treat GDM earlier in pregnancy to see if we can improve outcomes.

This work could not be done without an EHR. After all, the scale of the GDM investigation necessitated automation. How else could one assess the pregnancy outcomes of 10,000 women with GDM and link them to their children's weight five years later? The answer: only by having the medical records of 650,000 Kaiser Permanente members in the Pacific Northwest and Hawaii over a five-year period, reflecting 20 percent of the areas' populations; and only by having 26,211 subjects with GDM and without pre-existing diabetes. Only by having data for 9,439 pairs of mothers and children (who had weights recorded between ages five and seven).

Hillier's work demonstrates just one of the many ways that EHRs have supercharged research at Kaiser Permanente. Robust data gives ballast to population-based research, which now has larger, more representative sample sizes. It is now possible to work with data from 6,000 teens with depression, 10,000 people with end-stage chronic kidney disease, 45,000 women due for mammograms, 100,000 smokers, and 150,000 people with type 2 diabetes.

Not only is the data more comprehensive, but we can query databases at lightning speed. We can fine-tune randomization and recruitment targeting. Observational and cross-sectional studies have larger sample sizes. Prospective studies can draw from larger pools for recruitment and are able to find better matches of comparability between intervention and nonintervention cohorts. Participants represent a heterogeneous population of men and women of different ages, ethnic, racial, and socioeconomic backgrounds—not just in a theoretical setting, but in real-world practice.

We can now study rare diseases—or rare events—that would otherwise be impossible to detect at the population level. EHRs will empower us to search for and collect data on these rare diseases efficiently and comprehensively. An excellent example is amyotrophic lateral sclerosis (ALS), also called Lou Gehrig's disease, in which certain brain and spinal cord nerve cells slowly die. ALS occurs in only one to two cases per 100,000 population. But thanks to KP HealthConnect, we are able to combine the medical records from three Kaiser Permanente regions—the Northwest, Northern California, and Southern California—to create a registry of 6,000 people with ALS, an invaluable tool both for research and for quality improvement initiatives.

This new scale of capability has become available only within the last decade with our earlier regional EHRs, and the full research capabilities of the system-wide KP HealthConnect are just beginning to manifest.

Improving Patient Safety

As discussed in the previous chapter, KP HealthConnect has improved patient safety through the use of automated, on-screen alerts for preventing errors in prescribing or notifying care givers about the need for screening or lab work. In our Colorado region, Marsha Raebel, PharmD, has been at the forefront of research to maximize KP HealthConnect's utility through alerts in both laboratory monitoring and prescription orders, using the EHR to facilitate communication not just among physicians, but also between the lab and the pharmacy.

Lab monitoring is an essential part of long-term drug therapy for many patients, including people taking commonly prescribed medications like metformin (for diabetes), amiodarone (for arrhythmia), lithium (for bipolar disorder), and theophylline (for asthma). Without monitoring, these and other drugs can cause organ dysfunction and electrolyte imbalance, with lasting effects. Certainly the patient has an interest in remembering to visit the lab, but it is also the responsibility of care givers within the health care delivery system. To test the efficacy of EHR laboratory monitoring alerts, Raebel and her colleagues conducted a randomized trial of 9,139 patients undergoing drug therapy with fourteen drugs (Raebel and others, 2006). The researchers worked with physicians and pharmacists to develop monitoring guidelines, which were incorporated into a computerized alert system so that pharmacists were notified of missing laboratory results for those patients who were supposed to be monitored for drug therapy. The study's intervention included an electronic pharmacy alert when a prescription order was placed for a patient missing laboratory results. Following the alert, pharmacists would then order tests, remind patients to undergo tests, and review and manage abnormal results.

Raebel found that the alert increased the percentage of patients who received the intervention. Overall, with the intervention, 64 percent of patient-drug combinations were monitored, versus 58 percent without the intervention. Of the fourteen drug combinations studied, the intervention improved lab monitoring referrals for six drugs—including most dramatically for amiodarone (from 55 to 77 percent, with the intervention), theophylline (28 to 54 percent), and lithium (28 to 42 percent).

Raebel had used the EHR to deliver the intervention and track results, demonstrating that lab alerts can be effectively implemented, with good results within the system (fostering collaboration among physicians, lab, and pharmacy) as well as for patient safety. Of the 1,981 new laboratory tests ordered, 1,472 (74 percent) were completed; these revealed 181 serum drug concentrations outside the therapeutic range and 126 abnormal blood chemistries, hormone levels, and complete blood counts. Clearly, the research resulted in marked improvements in patient safety.

Following this study, Raebel and colleagues published findings on a compilation of six medication safety research projects at Kaiser Permanente-Colorado designed to decrease medication errors and improve patient outcomes. Using the electronic health records of more than 400,000 members, the researchers studied prescribing for patients who were elderly, pregnant, with impaired kidney function, and more. Five interventions were put into routine care, and every intervention reduced errors, resulting in more than 4,000 errors avoided during the research phases (Raebel and others, 2008).

Similarly, in Kaiser Permanente-Northwest, CHR's David Smith, MD, studied the effects of EHR alerts for contraindicated prescriptions among elderly patients (Smith and others, 2006). Raebel and Smith used the EHR as a research tool to capture data on pharmacy dispensings. In addition, they programmed information into the EHR so it could respond with an alert that flagged possible problems with physician prescription orders—recommending either laboratory monitoring or other medications if the requested medicine were inappropriate or contraindicated. Finally, they used the EHR as both a tool for implementation of the intervention and the record through which they could study its effectiveness.

Developing Tools to Evaluate Care Quality

Data captured through EHR-fueled research can be used to create risk assessment and modeling tools that help predict which patients need the most care. Such tools also help in designing early intervention programs to avoid or delay the onset of disease, as demonstrated by nephrologist Brian Lee and care management analyst Ken Forbes, who developed a predictive model for identifying and generating referrals for patients at risk for kidney failure in Kaiser Permanente's Hawaii region (see Chapter Five).

While risk assessment tools can improve patient care, they can also be used to assess and compare clinic or hospital performance and evaluate quality of care. Using EHR data on patient physiology and diagnosis, Gabriel Escobar, MD, from Kaiser Permanente-Northern California's DOR, developed and tested a risk adjustment tool to assess probability of hospital mortality—enabling groups of hospitals to compare practice differences (Escobar and others, 2008). Such assessments have been done using administrative data, but Escobar and his colleagues included pre-admission automated physiology and diagnosis data (including outpatient laboratory, diagnosis, and patients' previous hospitalization data) for more sensitive modeling. He led a retrospective cohort study of 409,305 hospital stays involving 259,699 patients hospitalized between January 2002 and June 2005 in seventeen hospitals to assess information on inpatient and thirty-day mortality. Collapsing thousands of International Classification of Disease codes into a convenient set of primary conditions, Escobar and his colleagues developed an algorithm with forty-one comorbidities into a single continuous variable to determine mortality.

EHR research allows us to study care delivery systems from many vantage points. We can evaluate patient outcomes or clinical services from an individual patient or a population-based perspective. With this knowledge, we can see how well or poorly our programs are working. We can compare our performance within the organization and against government standards. This level of scrutiny also allows us to move from a treatment model of health care delivery toward a prevention model.

As noted in Chapter Six, chronic care management programs can improve patient outcomes, yet the success of those programs can vary dramatically, depending on how the programs are implemented. Julie Schmittdiel, PhD, and her colleagues from DOR in Kaiser Permanente-Northern California used the EHR to evaluate the effectiveness of the region's Diabetes Care Management Program (Schmittdiel and others, 2009). They wanted to know whether they were treating the right cohort of diabetes patients. They also wanted to see whether the program was actually improving outcomes for enrollees. In an observational study, they assessed records for 179,249 diabetes patients both in and out of the care management program. The research revealed that, in fact, the program was not adhering to eligibility guidelines for its target population as effectively as it could. It found that 16 percent of its enrollees did not meet entry criteria.

At the same time, the study demonstrated that patients in the program showed only slightly more improvement for poorly controlled blood sugar and lipid levels than a set of matching patients who were not enrolled in care management. Overall, patients in Kaiser Permanente-Northern California showed significant improvement in all three risk factor levels over time whether or not they were in the program.

With this introspective research facilitated by retrospective EHR review, we were able to track progress against ourselves and evaluate a critical program that had the potential to improve patient outcomes.

Moving from Retrospective to Prospective Research

Much of the research made possible by EHRs to date has been retrospective and observational data-only studies, primarily because we have widespread access to such rich information. We look forward to new possibilities for prospective studies that incorporate interventions using KP HealthConnect.

In vaccine safety research, for example, this can take the form of real-time surveillance, which has been enabled just within the past several years and promises to be an invaluable public health asset. In this field, the leap from data-only, observational, retrospective studies to real-time surveillance is less complex than other forms of population-based research because we are looking to the EHR for very specific pieces of data that are more or less standardized across time and/or place.

When vaccine safety research began in the 1970s, data requests were simple and straightforward: Did the patient get a vaccine, and was there a negative response? We began our research through manual inspection of paper medical records. Research was expected to take years instead of days, and epic pandemics were not anticipated.

In the late 1990s, CHR conducted a two-year study of the influenza vaccine's impact on elderly persons in three large health plans—Kaiser Permanente-Northwest, HealthPartners, and Oxford Health Plans (Nordin and others, 2001). For the study's two influenza seasons, the vaccine reduced all causes of death and hospitalization for influenza and pneumonia (a well-established flu complication). Vaccination reduced all influenza-related hospitalizations by 20 percent in year one and by almost 25 percent in year two. On the basis of the findings, the authors recommended that all elderly persons get an annual influenza vaccine. While influential, these results took up to two years to analyze and publish.

The next transformation of vaccine research resulted from the 9/11 terrorist attacks. The threat of bioterrorism expedited the need to conduct real-time public health surveillance. Just a month after 9/11, in October 2001, the speed of EHR data evaluation was tested in the Kaiser Permanente-Mid-Atlantic States region, when three Kaiser Permanente members in Washington, D.C., were infected with anthrax. This began an intense rallying within the region (and among community and public health authorities) to coordinate and analyze massive amounts of patient data on infectious disease. At the time, a thousand entries were made in PACE, the region's pre–KP HealthConnect EHR, under HAZMAT notation shortly after the crisis broke (Stewart, 2002). This rapid and large-scale information processing not only enhanced patient safety but also demonstrated the utility of real-time surveillance in health crisis management. Soon the federal government put together multiple groups to conduct syndromic surveillance.

Meanwhile, as researchers foresaw the promise of automated data retrieval, they launched the Vaccine Safety Datalink (VSD) in 1990, a collaborative effort with the Centers for Disease Control to review medical records and monitor immunization safety. As the pace of public health protections quickened and the stakes and costs mounted, the VSD has taken up the charge for real-time surveillance. Among eight of its member organizations—which today include four Kaiser Permanente regions—VSD created its own virtual data warehouse to analyze EHR data on vaccines. VSD developed its own data retrieval, management processes, and statistical methods to handle the volume of data. Over the past several years, the VSD has successfully conducted real-time surveillance on a half-dozen newly licensed vaccines, including those for rotavirus, human papillomavirus, and H1N1 influenza. In one such study, the VSD identified a safety signal related to a new vaccine for children, which was reported to cause seizures. Once the signal was identified, it was thoroughly investigated and confirmed over the course of several months. The findings led to recommendations that have since changed how the vaccine is administered to young children. Without this real-time surveillance, identifying this signal would have taken at least a year—during which time more children would have experienced negative reactions to the vaccine.

Taking Data Gathering to a New Level

Real-time surveillance conducted by the VSD is now being adopted and applied by the Sentinel Initiative, a federal program launched in May 2008 by the Secretary of Health and Human Services and the Federal Drug Administration (FDA)

Commissioner to create a national electronic system for monitoring product safety. The Sentinel Initiative will draw on the capabilities of many existing automated health care data systems to augment the agency's current surveillance capabilities.

The VSD highlights the capabilities of immediate analysis of massive amounts of data. It is just one manifestation of data-sharing across health care delivery systems beyond Kaiser Permanente and one program of many within the Health Maintenance Organization Research Network. A consortium of fifteen HMO organizations (including six Kaiser Permanente regions), the network was formed in 1995 to take advantage of similar data and NIH interests that crossed organizations. The network has formal research and development programs with more than 250 researchers, 1,500 active research projects, and a population of more than fifteen million people. Resources include in-house survey research programs and research clinics, as well as standardized datasets.

Among the largest efforts of the HMO Research Network is the creation and implementation of the Virtual Data Warehouse (VDW), which will facilitate information exchange across all regions of Kaiser Permanente as well as inter-institutionally within the research network, greatly expanding these capabilities. The virtual data warehouse was started within the research network because every organization has its own data collection systems: its own EHR, hospital discharge abstract, claims, dispensing, membership, and tumor registry information. The goal of the virtual data warehouse is not to pool this data literally, but rather to harmonize its content for a common usage. Therefore, we are creating comparable datasets and formats, so while local data warehouse files are stored locally, queries may be run in parallel across multiple sites, sending back results (not data), protecting patient privacy and confidentiality.

To get a sense of scale, in Kaiser Permanente-Northern California, the local DOR data warehouse contains all aspects of clinical data dating from the early 1990s, including diagnostic, procedural, encounter, and pharmacy data. The DOR also combines patient demographic data, geocoding (through census data), laboratory use, mortality and cause of death from Kaiser Permanente records, state vital statistics, and federal Social Security data. Similarly, in Kaiser Permanente-Northwest, the CHR data warehouse stores more than 600 terabytes of data for multisite projects; creates standardized data files; builds risk assessment tools, pregnancy episode algorithms, and cancer counters; and gathers information from fourteen sources of diagnosis data, from home health to claims, from hospital discharge abstracts to new inpatient data. Amplify these capabilities many times over—across Kaiser Permanente research divisions and data warehouses of other members of the HMO Research Network—and the power of the virtual data warehouse becomes clear. With sixteen million electronic records, this virtual entity will become one of the largest repositories of public health data in the world.

Comparative Effectiveness Research

Until recently, the virtual data warehouse was a concept; today, it is the platform for Kaiser Permanente's organization-wide comparative effectiveness research. Comparative effectiveness research is objective scientific inquiry to determine the most clinically successful and cost-effective treatment for patients, without influence from parties with a financial interest. It is needed precisely because the FDA is not set up to compare one treatment, drug, or procedure with another, but only to make drug approval decisions based on tests of safety and efficacy against a placebo.

Kaiser Permanente recently launched the Center for Effectiveness and Safety Research, which enables us to conduct large-scale studies to help advance public health. A stellar example of this type of research arose out of Kaiser Permanente-Northern California's DOR, which conducted a joint study with the FDA on Vioxx (Graham and others, 2005). Studying the EHRs of 1.39 million Kaiser Permanente members, researchers compared the outcomes of 40,405 patients taking Celebrex to those of 26,748 patients taking Vioxx. Researchers found that sudden cardiac deaths and heart attack rates tripled for patients taking Vioxx compared with those taking the rival drug. When the results were released in September 2004, the manufacturer took its $2.5 billion-a-year pain drug, Vioxx, off the market.

KP HealthConnect will allow us to take such comparative effectiveness research to new and more complex levels. A prime example is research now under way in four Kaiser Permanente regions on the treatment of late-stage cancer. Debra Ritzwoller, PhD, of Kaiser Permanente-Colorado's Institute for Health Research, is leading a team of investigators in new work to build data infrastructure to support comparative effectiveness studies of treatment for late-stage cancers and to support studies of patterns of care and outcomes among patients with advanced cancer.

Using the power of KP HealthConnect, the researchers are delving deep into complex, multilayered information to develop, validate, and implement care strategies. They will follow particular treatment regimens and analyze patterns of care, from the use of chemotherapy to use and frequency of high-cost imaging. This research will be used to identify the best treatments for physicians to follow and provide the tools to allow them to track how well they work for individual patients.

While this work may have been possible before KP HealthConnect, it certainly would have taken much longer and have been much more costly.

Personalized Medicine, Genetics, and Genomics

During the past decade, genetic research has given scientists new tools with which to understand, diagnose, treat, and prevent disease. In recent years, genomic and other molecular tests have been recommended for cancer treatment to identify individuals at high risk, screen and perform early detection, identify prognostic markers, and guide courses of therapy. Researchers will soon discover genetic factors that allow us to improve our predictions regarding other health risks, such as addiction, obesity, diabetes, heart disease, depression, and much more. With newfound understanding of genetics and genomics, we are entering the realm of personalized medicine, in which researchers and physicians will create tailor-made treatment plans designed for a patient's specific genome.

In Kaiser Permanente-Northwest, CHR's Katrina Goddard, PhD, and Evelyn Whitlock, MD, MPH, with partners Lawrence Kushi, ScD, from Kaiser Permanente-Northern California's DOR, and members of the Cancer Research Network (also a part of the HMO Research Network) have been funded to compare the effectiveness of genetic tests for colon cancer risk prediction and treatment. Where historically we have prescribed largely via trial and error, now drug and treatment plans may be guided by genomic and genetic information nested within the EHR. This information will travel with the patient throughout his or her lifetime.

Similar farsighted plans are under way at DOR in Kaiser Permanente-Northern California. Kaiser Permanente's Research Program on Genes, Environment, and Health (RPGEH), led by Catherine Schaefer, PhD, launched in February 2007 and will soon reach its goal of building a world-class genetic epidemiology resource, one of the largest biorepositories to facilitate research on how genes and the environment affect health. Nearly 400,000 Kaiser Permanente-Northern California members have voluntarily completed the RPGEH health survey and approximately 70,000 have already contributed saliva samples for the biorepository.

We now recognize the power of EHRs to advance knowledge in ways we would not have imagined when we first started research at Kaiser Permanente more than half a century ago. We nonetheless have challenges ahead, particularly questions around the proprietary nature of patient data. As the Virtual Data Warehouse develops and becomes a reality through the Center for Effectiveness and Safety Research, Kaiser Permanente patient data continues to be segmented by region. Because each region has different data needs and practices, discrete databases continue as an issue within the organization. But the more we refine the virtual warehouse, the closer we get to seamless analysis across the system.

While the VDW promises to knit together discrete region-specific data platforms, there is room for further development of disease-specific registries in each region, following the model of Kaiser Permanente Colorado's research institute, which has dozens of registries in its HealthTrac system. Kaiser Permanente Northern California's research division also has rich registry information, dating from its Multiphasic Health Checkup, begun in 1964, and the Member Health Survey, started in 1993, as well as cancer, HIV, diabetes, and neonatal registries. Expansion of registries offers tremendous potential, particularly with advancements in genetic research and given the automated nature of data processing, organization, and management that registries would require.

Tapping New Data Sources: Natural Language Processing and Patient-Entered Data

Another area for EHR research is natural language processing, which can be used to extract data from free-text portions of the EHR. It is estimated that about half of the patient information assessing health, care, and quality within the EHR is coded, while the other half is qualitative free text embedded in the physician's notes, which cannot be summarized with traditional automated methods. As shown by the first case study at the end of this chapter, natural language processing provides new automated methods with the potential to unleash the 50 percent of the information within a medical record that remains inaccessible to us today, bringing it out of the shadows of unusable free text into the coded world of automated summary in the EHR.

Just as free-text notations contain critical health data, so do patients themselves. The utility of the EHR can be limited by poor or inadequate patient-physician communication, but this can be remedied by including patients in the information-gathering process. Greater patient participation in and ownership of electronic medical information can boost the richness and accuracy of EHRs. This area holds great potential as patients become increasingly computer literate and technology continues to offer an impressive array of validated instruments to enhance EHR information. Web-based questionnaires that feed into the EHR and the panel support tool help clinicians incorporate subjective information that may not come up in an office visit, particularly in areas such as pediatrics, psychiatry, and chronic condition management.

Three EHR-Enabled Research Case Studies

Following are summaries of three additional Kaiser Permanente research studies—selected from among hundreds of good examples—that illustrate how EHR-enabled research is being quickly translated into improved patient care and better health outcomes.

Turning Physicians' Free-Text Notations into Computer-Readable Data

As a physician attends to the patient during an office visit, he or she records details of the visit in KP HealthConnect in two ways: by navigating a point-and-click environment of clinical options with a mouse, which translates selections into coded data in the electronic record, and by making free-text notations using traditional clinical narratives. Preventive care, family history, and counseling are all examples of information particularly rich in free-text notations because they involve complex discussion between providers and patients that cannot be easily coded.

It is estimated that the patient information in an electronic record is distributed about equally between both methods of natural language note-taking and coded data capture. While the coded data can be automatically summarized by analysts using traditional database tools, the free-text notation cannot be "translated" or summarized in this way. What this means is that half of the information needed for comprehensive care quality assessment is not available through computerized analysis methods, which seriously limits the utility of EHRs.

To address these limitations, Kaiser Permanente researchers in the Northwest region created an experimental natural language processing computer system called MediClass, which automatically processes both the coded and free-text portions of electronic records that pertain to evidence-based care for a particular condition.

To test the accuracy of their system, the researchers configured MediClass to process all coded and natural language information relevant to the evidence-based care model for providing smoking cessation treatment (Hazlehurst and others, 2005). They focused on smoking cessation first because it requires physician counseling, which is recorded in free-text notes, and because of the clinical significance of smoking.

In smoking cessation counseling, physicians use a process known as the "5As"—Ask about smoking status; Advise users to quit; Assess willingness to quit; Assist patients' efforts through treatment or referrals; and Arrange follow-up. Using the same medical records, the study compared the performance of MediClass to that of human coders, who were trained to read and abstract specific data relevant to the 5As from the same set of medical records. They processed five hundred primary care encounter records from the electronic databases of four different health plans, including three Kaiser Permanente regions, and found that in 91 percent of the cases, MediClass agreed with the majority opinions of the human coders in deciphering free-text information relevant to the 5As. Furthermore, the researchers reported that, once installed, a natural language processing system such as MediClass is more than a hundred times faster than trained human data abstractors, and the total cost is negligible.

The Center for Health Research suggests that natural language processing may in effect double the amount of information available in EHRs that could be used to improve patient care and treatment.

Reducing the Overuse of Antibiotic Treatment for Viruses

Although viruses do not respond to antibiotic treatment, physicians nonetheless prescribe these medications to about half of all patients with colds and upper respiratory infections, and up to 80 percent of patients with bronchitis. Such overuse has been implicated in the emergence and spread of antibiotic-resistant bacteria, particularly *Streptococcus pneumoniae*, which is the leading bacterial cause of community-acquired pneumonia, meningitis, and otitis media in the United States.

To help reduce inappropriate antibiotic prescribing, Kaiser Permanente's Institute for Health Research conducted an intervention to educate patients and physicians about antibiotic overuse (Gonzales and others, 1999). Investigators used data from the pre–KP HealthConnect EHR during a four-month period over two successive years to assess the effect of the intervention on antibiotic prescription rates for patients diagnosed with uncomplicated bronchitis. The first year had no intervention. The second year involved a full intervention that consisted of printed materials on antibiotics and colds, flu, and bronchitis mailed to patients of one primary care clinic, as well as clinic office posters on the inappropriate use of antibiotics. In addition, the intervention taught clinic providers about evidence-based management of bronchitis and how to say "no" to patient requests for antibiotics. Two clinics served as control sites without any interventions, and another clinic received only educational posters.

Using highly specific data from the EHR, researchers matched antibiotic prescriptions to patient office visits that resulted in diagnoses of bronchitis at each of the four clinics. The study found that prescription rates at all four clinics were similar during the first year of the study; but at the clinic receiving the intervention, the prescribing rate dropped from 74 percent to 48 percent. Furthermore, the EHR data showed that return office visits within thirty days for either bronchitis or pneumonia remained consistent throughout the study, demonstrating that the reduced level of antibiotic prescriptions did not expose more members to bacterial respiratory infections.

In this way, EHR-based research was able to prove a hypothesis that could change antibiotic prescribing patterns in cold and flu season—which in turn could benefit public health by combating new patterns of antibiotic-resistant bacteria.

The Prevention Index, Generating Better Quality Measures

When Tom Vogt, MD, of Kaiser Permanente's Center for Health Research, saw KP HealthConnect coming online in Hawaii, he thought creatively about how best to make use of it. He wanted the EHR to be helpful not just in the physician's office but more broadly as a care delivery tool that would answer an expansive question: How well was Kaiser Permanente-Hawaii delivering preventive care services—not just individually but across clinics, the region, and even system-wide?

Vogt developed what he called the Prevention Index, a new and highly precise way to determine how many members were receiving appropriately timed screening for any number of conditions, as recommended by the U.S. Preventive Services Task Force (Vogt and others, 2004). Using a "person time" approach, the Prevention Index measured the precise proportion of time that individuals were below, at, or above recommended treatment goals.

The EHR already contained all the data the Prevention Index needed for its calculations. Vogt then developed an algorithm that assigned different weights to preventive services, depending on their relative health importance. The EHR-enabled Prevention Index was systematic and inexpensive, addressed various flaws of current quality measures, and included all prevention services rated as effective by consensus groups. It also facilitated delivery of precisely targeted interventions to improve care according to evidence-based guidelines, and it determined the relationship of guideline adherence to morbidity, mortality, and cost outcomes. It was driven by data already in the EHR.

Once the Prevention Index tool was developed, Vogt put it to work in 2005. Focusing on the years 1999–2002, he used a pre–KP HealthConnect EHR to study how well KP-Hawaii delivered ten preventive care services—through twenty medical offices with nearly eight hundred physicians and four hundred allied health care providers (Vogt and others, 2007). Preventive services included mammography, pneumococcal and influenza vaccines, tobacco status/counseling, and screening for Chlamydia, lipids, osteoporosis, cervical cancer, blood pressure, and colorectal cancer.

Use of the index revealed that, overall, about 47 percent of the eligible "person time" for all preventive services was provided as recommended in 2002. However, Vogt found wide ranges in coverage for specific services, from 19 percent for Chlamydia screening to 79.9 percent for blood pressure. He also found variation at the practice level, which swung from 3.3 percent to 99.6 percent for mammography screening.

The sensitivity and precision of the Prevention Index proved far more discerning than HEDIS scores and, as a result, more valuable in discovering areas for either emulation or improvement—in individual patient care, larger clinic or regional practice, or both. The Index could be expanded to areas of chronic disease management involving treatment to target physiologic levels, such as lipids, glycemic control, and blood pressure. So, in many ways, Vogt's Prevention Index, driven by EHR data, improved patient outcomes and quality of care delivery.

Conclusion

EHRs have transformed the research landscape. Just within the past several years, KP HealthConnect has become fully functioning and data-populated system-wide. Our research using this data has helped us improve patient safety, quality of care, and chronic disease management; prompted us to invest in further refinements to maximize the EHR's utility as a research resource; and given us an objective gauge to set better and more meaningful quality and care delivery standards both within Kaiser Permanente and at the national level. As we continue to pursue this research, we are also mastering new ways of using EHRs in research that will further advance public health—including real-time surveillance, comparative effectiveness research, and personalized medicine.

These endeavors will enable us to track and compare treatments, drugs, and devices to show what works and what doesn't. They will link care delivery to costs and mobilize translational medicine, so we can move discoveries from the laboratory into real-world clinical practice at a faster pace. We are just now approaching the time when we can fold genetic information into the EHR so it can inform treatment on an individualized basis. We will soon be able to conduct clinical trials using real-time surveillance, with immediate results that can improve patient health and safety and care delivery and efficiency.

This is a time of unprecedented opportunity in health research. We are poised to elevate the role of science as a force for positive change. We have new tools and technology—KP HealthConnect being a prime example—with limitless power and potential to advance human health.

SECTION FOUR

FUTURE DIRECTIONS

CHAPTER ELEVEN

KP HEALTHCONNECT AND THE ARCHIMEDES MODEL

A Step into the Future of Health Care

By David M. Eddy, MD, PhD

Chapter Summary

This chapter describes how linking an electronic health record such as KP HealthConnect to a powerful new physiology-based, clinically accurate, computerized simulation model known as the Archimedes Model, can improve the quality and efficiency of health care. The Archimedes Model, developed by the author and his colleague Len Schlessinger and sponsored by Kaiser Permanente, provides a means of simulating clinical trials that are impractical to conduct in the real world, and evaluating a variety of programs and policies that are vital to improving health care quality and costs. By linking the model to KP HealthConnect's wealth of patient-specific and population data, the model can create a virtual world in which the time and cost constraints of real-world health care studies are overcome to arrive at highly reliable conclusions to support clinical and operational decision making. The author describes how the model has been validated in numerous studies comparing the results of Archimedes's simulated trials to those of real-world clinical trials, and how the linkage of Archimedes to KP HealthConnect could soon provide answers to some of the most vital problems confronting health care.

David M. Eddy, MD, PhD, was responsible for the initiation and medical development of the Archimedes Model, with the sponsorship of Kaiser Permanente. He has been a long-time consultant to Kaiser Permanente and is a member of the Institute of Medicine/National Academy of Science.

Introduction

Kaiser Permanente HealthConnect, as it exists today, provides great value and is an enormous improvement over the paper system it replaced. It collects, stores, retrieves, and displays longitudinal, person-specific data on all the relevant aspects of patient care. Although its primary purpose is to facilitate the care of individual patients, the data in KP HealthConnect can be used to perform many other functions, such as calculating a wide variety of measures of performance and quality, identifying patients indicated for interventions and outreach programs, and creating a picture of the past and current states of the Kaiser Permanente population. KP HealthConnect also has the ability to support decisions by flagging various events and passing messages to clinicians on how to manage those events.

Linking KP HealthConnect to a model like Archimedes can add substantially to its value by significantly enhancing a critical step in the quality improvement cycle—the analysis of data to inform decisions about the best ways to provide care. KP HealthConnect by itself has tools for filtering and organizing raw data about all the pertinent clinical events that occur throughout Kaiser Permanente and displaying in more meaningful form information about individual patients, populations, and the delivery system as a whole. But whereas KP HealthConnect can describe what happened, Archimedes is designed to determine why it happened and the quantitative relationships between various factors. It is also designed to answer questions about the expected effects of new options that might be considered for improving the system—questions that electronic health records (EHRs) on their own are powerless to address.

Why a Mathematical Model Is Needed

Traditionally, it was generally assumed that decisions about patient care could and should be left to individual physicians. However, over the past three decades numerous studies have shown that this was not a safe assumption. These studies revealed that physicians displayed wide ranges of uncertainty about the outcomes of the tests and treatments they were recommending. They varied widely in their beliefs about what tests and treatments should be done to particular patients. There were wide variations in their practices. And as judged by their peers, there were high rates of inappropriate care. These discoveries have raised serious doubts about the quality of care (for example, McGlynn and others, 2003).

Over the same period, payers of health care have become more and more troubled by the cost of care, which is pushing aside other priorities for families, businesses, states, and the federal government. These two forces—questionable quality and rising costs—led to the development of a large number of clinical management tools designed to improve quality and control costs. They include evidence-based guidelines; performance measurement; disease management; physician payment incentive programs based on quality and outcomes; comparative effectiveness programs for drugs, devices, and other treatments; and other quality and cost containment programs. As a result, more and more decisions are being made, or at least guided, at higher levels in health care organizations by expert committees for quality improvement, clinical guidelines, drug formularies, and approval of new technologies. Policies and programs designed by these and other committees require much more rigorous quantitative analysis than was required in the past.

More Complex Questions—Some Examples

The complexity of today's decisions is best appreciated through some examples.

For instance, let us say a pharmaceutical company has just introduced a new drug. In clinical trials it is slightly more effective than the current drug (and/or has a slightly lower rate of side effects), but it costs more. Should we add it to the formulary? If so, for which patients should it be indicated? If we have a tiered payment system, which tier should it be in? If we want to add a co-payment, how much should it be? If the drug is used in the patients for whom it appears to be indicated, how will that affect quality? How many complications of the disease or side effects will it prevent? How will it affect the pharmacy budget? To what extent will the increased pharmacy costs be offset by preventing complications of the disease and side effects? If there is an offset, how long will it take for the drug to pay for itself?

Another example: a health care organization notices that its physicians vary widely in the schedules they use for following up with patients who have chronic conditions. Some are asking to see their patients on a monthly basis while others are content to wait six months. They also vary widely in the tests they are using. Taking into account the clinical outcomes and the costs of visits and tests, how important are these variations? What would be the effect on cost and quality if we could convert high users of care to become low users?

Or, let us say a health plan wants to focus more on prevention. What should it focus on: Obesity? Smoking? Tighter control of cholesterol or blood pressure? Aspirin use? Diet and exercise? For each of these there are a variety of different programs, such as different strategies for reducing obesity or getting people to stop smoking. They have different intensities, cost different amounts of money, and make different claims about success rates. Which should be used? For example, if a particular smoking cessation program has a one-year quit rate of 15 percent but costs $50 per smoker, while another has a one-year quit rate of 10 percent but costs $15, which will be the best use of resources? Will the higher costs of the more expensive program be offset by savings from preventing cardiovascular disease and cancer?

Questions can also be asked at the level of individual physicians and patients. For example, take Mrs. Smith. Her doctor knows she is fifty-eight years old; has had diabetes since she was forty-five; and is treated with metformin, with a current hemoglobin A1c level of 7.2 percent (a measure of blood sugar control). He also knows lots of other clinically relevant information about her, including her family history. What is her chance of a heart attack, stroke, retinopathy, foot ulcer, or other outcome in the next five years? Ten years? Lifetime? What would be the effects on each of these outcomes of various treatments, such as trying harder to get her A1c level below 7, getting her to lose weight, lowering her LDL cholesterol, or lowering her blood pressure? Which of these treatments is most important? Is there an optimal combination of treatments?

Ideally, questions like these would be answered with empirical studies such as controlled clinical trials and demonstration programs. However, this is not feasible. Even one clinical trial can cost tens—sometimes hundreds—of millions of dollars and require many years to design, set up, conduct, and analyze. Depending on the nature of the question, data on thousands of patients can be required. By the time the study was complete, there may well be new tests, treatments, or evidence that make the trial's results obsolete, or that simply raise more questions. When the full range of questions and all of the different variations and options within those questions are taken into consideration, the impossibility of answering them all with empirical studies is clear. But the questions do not go away. One way or another, questions will be answered and decisions will be made. Even a decision to avoid a question is a decision.

The future of health care rests squarely on how well health care organizations can answer these types of questions. Each has huge leverage for affecting both quality and cost, and each requires quantitative methods that take into account the actual magnitudes of the benefits, harm, and costs. Without knowing the magnitudes of those outcomes it is not possible to make comparisons, set priorities, or determine the best way to use limited resources to maximize quality. It is no insult to anyone to say that questions like these are too complicated for the unaided human mind. Today's questions require more powerful tools.

Why EHRs Cannot Answer These Questions

EHRs like KP HealthConnect can provide a great deal of information that was never accessible with paper-based systems. But there is a limit to what they can do. Most important, they only contain information about the present and the past. If the only questions we want to ask are about what is happening now or about what happened in the past, KP HealthConnect can answer them.

However, the questions we need to answer are not about the past or even about the present, but are about what we should do in the future. And the constant expansion of medical knowledge and technologies means that if we are interested in anything beyond the next year or two, the future is not a straight-line projection from the past. After all, an EHR can contain no longitudinal data about the effects of new tests or treatments, simply because they are new. It can answer questions only about tests and treatments that have been in use for at least the time period of interest.

Even for tests and treatments that have been in use for the time period of interest, there are other factors that limit the types of questions that can be answered. Suppose that the drugs we want to compare are both old and we can find two groups of people who were treated with the different drugs. Before we can compare the outcomes in those two groups and draw conclusions about the effectiveness of the drugs, we need to ensure that those who were treated with the old drug and the new drug were similar in all other ways that might affect their chances of the outcomes of interest. This is very unlikely, given the great variety in risk factors for most serious conditions. If the patients in the two groups were treated differently for any particular conditions, we would not be able to determine if any difference in outcomes was due to the superiority of one drug over the other rather than other differences in treatment.

This and other problems become more and more difficult as the number of options to be explored increases and the differences between options become more subtle. Examples are different criteria for identifying patients indicated for treatment, different dosages of drugs, different treatment targets, different ways to sequence tests or treatments, different follow-up protocols, and so forth.

Health services researchers have developed risk-adjustment methods to try to overcome these problems, but they would be the first to admit that those methods still leave a wide range of uncertainty around the answers. They are useful for evaluating programs that have been launched on a relatively large scale and introduced relatively "cleanly," but these methods become more and more limited when they are asked to determine the effects of subtle differences in treatments, and they are useless for evaluating new tests and treatments or new uses of tests and treatments that are not in the EHR dataset at all.

To summarize, an EHR is invaluable for observing what happened in the past and what is happening now, but it is not good for determining what will happen in the future, what would happen if we did something differently, or the merits of different options.

The Role of Mathematical Models

An EHR such as KP HealthConnect can be made more powerful by linking it to a simulation model like Archimedes, where by "link" we mean use the data in KP HealthConnect to improve and tune the model, and then use the model to answer the questions needed for decision making. The use of models in this fashion is not new. When Boeing designs a new airplane, it faces scores of questions about the design of the wing, shape of the body, weight, engine power, and other variables. It does not build prototypes of all the possible combinations, fly them, and get the pilots' assessments. That would be impossibly time-consuming and expensive. Boeing uses the principles of physics and data from wind tunnels to build mathematical representations of the planes and then flies the virtual plane inside a computer. Boeing does conduct experiments. But the purpose of any particular experiment is not so much to get an answer to one particular question as it is to collect data to build models that can answer hundreds of questions.

Virtually every other sector of our economy uses mathematical models to manage complexity and uncertainty. Architects use them to design buildings, engineers use them to calculate the trajectories of satellites, UPS uses them to calculate optimal transportation routes, and Intel uses them to design its chips. The idea of using data from EHRs to build models and then use the models to answer a variety of questions has a long history of successes. There is little question that, over time, they will play a larger and larger role in health care, and linking KP HealthConnect to the Archimedes Model is an excellent place to start.

Types of Models

Data from a comprehensive EHR such as KP HealthConnect, along with other sources, can be used to help build a wide variety of models. At one end of the spectrum, in terms of simplicity, are single equation models such as regression equations to help adjust for confounding factors ("risk adjustment") or "predictive models" to help project a patient's costs for the coming year on the basis of what happened in recent past years. Both of these are common, generally well-accepted types of models but of limited value.

However, if we want to answer the types of questions listed earlier in this chapter, we need a model that is built at the same level of "clinical realism" as the questions that are being asked. Ideally, the model should encompass all the biological variables that physicians consider to be important in the management of their patients, and it should relate them to one another and to health outcomes in a natural way. This level of detail is also needed to make the model credible to clinicians. It must span all types of interventions (primary prevention, screening, diagnosis, treatment, secondary prevention, and support care) and span multiple diseases using the same methodology. A broad span is also required to address patients who have multiple diseases (comorbidities), syndromes that affect multiple organ systems, drugs that have multiple effects, and combinations of drugs. It must also function in continuous time and be able to address events that can change as rapidly as minute-by-minute, or as slowly as years. Finally, to be credible, a model should be able to simulate the most important epidemiological studies and clinical trials and match or predict their results within the appropriate confidence limits.

The Archimedes Model

The Archimedes Model was designed to be as clinically realistic as possible with current knowledge and to address the types of questions listed earlier. At the center of the model is a set of ordinary and differential equations that represent physiological pathways at the "organ" level (Schlessinger and Eddy, 2002; Eddy and Schlessinger, 2003a). This is roughly the same level of detail at which clinicians think, including the same types of risk factors, physiological variables, tests, treatments, and outcomes that appear in patient charts and the design of clinical trials. At the time of this writing, the model includes pathways relating to diabetes; congestive heart failure; coronary artery disease; stroke; hypertension; obesity; metabolic syndrome; asthma; and prevention and screening of cancers of the lung, breast, and colon, in a single integrated model. Other conditions are being added as time and resources permit.

The model also includes equations that represent the development and progression of diseases, occurrence of signs and symptoms; patient behaviors in seeking care and complying with treatments; care processes and protocols; clinical events such as office visits and admissions; tests and treatments; physician behaviors and performance; logistics and utilization, such as emergency department visits, admissions, and procedures; costs; and measures of quality of life.

Because the model uses differential equations to represent physiology and diseases, time is continuous, biological variables are continuously interacting, any event can occur at any time, and the timing of events is as condensed or drawn out as occurs in reality. Clinical outcomes are defined in terms of the underlying variables. Because the model includes underlying physiological variables, it is able to incorporate different definitions and changes in definitions. The effects of interventions are modeled at the level of the underlying biology. The inclusion of multiple organ systems and diseases as part of a single physiology enables more accurate representation of the effects of syndromes, comorbidities, multiple drugs, and drugs with multiple effects.

The Archimedes Model was formulated and programmed so that it can be expanded, deepened, and updated with relative ease. It is modularized so that parts of the model can be added or changed without requiring reprogramming of other modules. This enables the addition of new conditions, tests, and treatments, as well as updating the model. The modularization is hierarchical, enabling Archimedes scientists to build deeper layers of clinical and physiological realism as needed to address specific questions. The model runs on a grid of computers using distributed computing methods.

The model is also constructed so that it can be tailored to different settings—different populations, such as age, sex, race/ethnicity, behaviors, risk factors, and incidence rates; different care processes and levels of performance; and different costs. Examples of possible settings are the United States, the state of California, Kaiser Permanente and any of its regions, the employees of a major company, or patients covered by Medicare.

Validation Tests

The Archimedes Model is validated by using it to simulate epidemiological studies and controlled clinical trials and then comparing the model's predicted or calculated results against the real results.

An example is the simulation of the Heart Protection Study, which consisted of men and women between forty and eighty years of age who had had a previous myocardial infarction or who currently (at the time of the trial) had had a bypass graft or angioplasty. Data included aggregated information on such things as the proportion of patients who had had a myocardial infarction, the proportion who had diabetes, the average HDL level, and other variables typically found in a table of baseline characteristics. The trial had two arms, with one half of the population being given simvastatin 40 mg and the other half receiving usual care but without simvastatin. The trial measured fatal and nonfatal myocardial infarctions and strokes.

The real trial, as well as the virtual trial conducted within Archimedes, had a sample size of 20,000 people, was conducted over a five-year time period, and reported Kaplan-Meier curves. The results of the simulated trial and the results of the actual trial are compared in Figure 11.1.

Thus far, more than a dozen epidemiological studies and approximately fifty controlled clinical trials have been simulated and the results validated. The first seventy-four validation exercises involving eighteen clinical trials have been published (Eddy and Schlessinger, 2003b). There is an ongoing process of validating the model against the landmark trials relating to the conditions and diseases included in the model. In addition, for particular projects the Archimedes team works with the organizations sponsoring the trials to identify clinical trials and other studies needed to document the model's accuracy for those particular applications. Recently, the model's accuracy in predicting events in realistic settings has been tested in Kaiser Permanente (described later in this chapter). The model is periodically revalidated against a suite of landmark trials every time the model is extended, deepened, or upgraded on the basis of new science, technology, or evidence. These validations check the model's accuracy and build confidence in its results.

Linking Archimedes to KP HealthConnect Data

The Archimedes Model draws on data from many different sources—epidemiological data; the effects of demographics, risk factors, and behaviors on the occurrence and progression of diseases; basic science studies for various aspects of physiology such as heart function; basic clinical studies for such things as physiological pathways, occurrence of symptoms, and accuracies of tests; and controlled clinical trials. All this data is used to help build and validate the model.

FIGURE 11.1. COMPARISON OF SIMULATED ARCHIMEDES TRIAL TO REAL TRIAL FOR THE HEART PROTECTION STUDY.

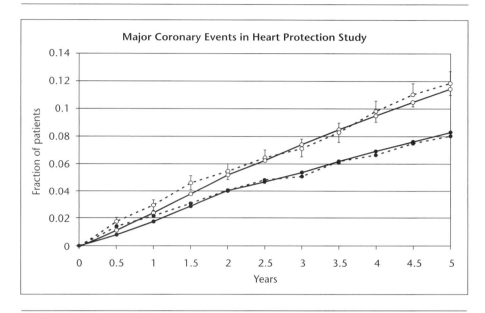

The two upper lines represent the simulated trial (dotted line) and the real trial (solid line) for the control group; the lower lines represent the simulated versus real trial for the treated group.

However, there are two critically important parts of medical practice that these sources do not provide information on. The first pertains to individual variations in the progression of diseases, for which person-specific longitudinal data from realistic settings is needed. The second pertains to the settings in which health care is delivered. This is important because the effects of an intervention can depend as much on the particular setting in which it is delivered as on the intervention itself. To be most accurate in a particular setting, the model should be calibrated using data gathered from that setting to match its population, care processes, utilization, and costs.

This is precisely the type of information KP HealthConnect provides. This person-specific and setting-specific data enables not only an accurate representation of the health care organization as a whole but accurate representations of particular regions, or even particular medical centers within regions.

Example: Simulating a Diabetes Intervention in Kaiser Permanente. Six years ago, some physicians at Kaiser Permanente came up with an idea: What if Kaiser

Permanente's members with diabetes were systematically given a bundle of drugs consisting of aspirin, lovastatin (a cholesterol drug), and lisinopril (a blood pressure drug)—nicknamed "A-L-L." Their clinical intuition told them that it should have an important effect on complications of diabetes. However, there was no direct evidence of that and no way to determine the magnitude of the effects on either clinical outcomes or costs. They knew they needed this type of information if they were to convince the organization to adopt the program, or even conduct a trial to test it. They decided to use the Archimedes Model to predict the expected outcomes.

To analyze this problem, an Archimedes team created a simulated population that represented the people with diabetes in Kaiser Permanente. The team also used information on Kaiser Permanente's costs for drugs, lab tests, office visits, and admissions for heart attacks and strokes, for which diabetes is a major risk factor. The team then created two scenarios to represent alternative management strategies for patients with diabetes. In one scenario, called "current care," virtual patients with diabetes continued to receive the type of care they had been receiving in the past, based on national guidelines with realistic levels of performance and compliance. In the other scenario, called "A-L-L regimen," virtual patients with diabetes were given the A-L-L regimen in addition to current care. The team then used the Archimedes Model to forecast the health, logistic, and economic outcomes for both scenarios over a thirty-year period, with measurements at annual intervals.

The Archimedes Model predicted that, when added to current care, the A-L-L regimen should reduce heart attacks and strokes by approximately 71 percent and should reduce diabetes-related costs by approximately $500 per person per year. The model predicted that the effect on health outcomes would begin almost immediately, within the first two years. The effect on costs was estimated to be slower in developing, with savings of approximately $350 per person in the initial years, but gradually increasing to more than $700 per person per year. On the basis of this analysis, Kaiser Permanente decided to launch and heavily promote a program-wide effort to provide the A-L-L regimen to all patients with diabetes. The program was begun in 2004.

Three years later, Kaiser Permanente's Care Management Institute (CMI) conducted an independent evaluation to determine the extent to which the A-L-L regimen was being used, and the regimen's actual effects on the incidence of cardiovascular disease (Dudl and others, 2009). During 2004 and 2005, approximately 28 percent of people with diabetes were receiving the A-L-L regimen at a low intensity (approximately less than half the intended compliance rate) and 13 percent were receiving the regimen at a high intensity (more than half the intended compliance rate). CMI calculated that by the third year of implementation, in 2006, admissions for heart attacks and strokes had decreased by 60 percent in people receiving low intensity of the A-L-L regimen, and were virtually eliminated in people receiving the A-L-L regimen at high intensity. The study concluded that the results were consistent with those modeled by Archimedes.

In absolute terms, CMI estimated that A-L-L prevented 1,271 hospitalizations for heart attacks and strokes in 2006 in the population of about 68,560 members with diabetes exposed to the A-L-L regimen. They estimated that if projected to the entire Kaiser Permanente diabetes population, more than 8,000 hospitalizations for heart attacks and strokes would be prevented each year. CMI also estimated a net savings (after paying for the costs of the three drugs) of more than $28 million a year in those exposed to A-L-L, or approximately $440 per person with diabetes. Projected across the entire Kaiser Permanente diabetes population, the savings would be approximately $175 million a year. On the basis of this, Kaiser Permanente has decided to intensify its efforts to deliver the A-L-L regimen to the remainder of its diabetic population.

This example took place before KP HealthConnect was fully implemented, using some data from an earlier EHR. Nonetheless it is a good example of the type of analysis that can be done by linking data from an EHR to the Archimedes Model. KP HealthConnect provides data on the setting, including the population, care processes, current levels of use of the drugs, and costs. Archimedes then simulates what would happen if the proposed interventions were actually implemented. The results of the simulation provide decision makers with information that would otherwise never have been available. Given the high degree of financial and clinical commitment required to implement a program such as A-L-L, the program might never have been implemented without the projections from the Archimedes Model. Data from KP Health-Connect were then used to conduct an evaluation to confirm the projections and the success of the program. This cycle can continue with additional refinements to the A-L-L protocol.

Example: Individualized Guidelines. Guidelines are an indispensible part of medical practice. Their main role is to assist physician decisions by condensing extremely complex problems into simple rules of thumb. Despite their value, guidelines have shortcomings. One of the most important is that, as described earlier, they are often very simplistic and clinically unrealistic. They tend to focus on one factor at a time (for example, blood pressure) and they tend to use sharp cut points to separate those who should be treated from those who should not.

This raises an obvious question: What could be gained if we tried to tailor guidelines more closely to each patient's specific needs? We call this approach "individualized guidelines" to distinguish them from guidelines as they are currently designed, which we will call "traditional" or "population-based" guidelines. Individualized guidelines consider each person one-by-one, take into account all the pertinent characteristics and risk factors for that person, identify all the interventions from which that person might benefit, calculate the expected improvement in health outcomes for each intervention one-by-one and in combination, and tailor the choice of interventions to optimize the benefit to each person.

Individualized guidelines can be created for each person using a tool based on the Archimedes Model. The tool can take into account information on more than forty variables relating to demographics, behaviors, biomarkers, health history, and current medications. The number of variables pertinent to any particular individual varies, but is typically fifteen to twenty-five and corresponds to the same variables a physician would evaluate in the routine care of a patient. The tool uses the information to calculate the individual's risk of a cardiovascular event, to identify all the potential treatments from which the patient might benefit, to calculate the degree of benefit that would be achieved if the patient took each one of the treatments one-by-one or in various combinations, and to calculate an overall "benefit score" that represents the benefit of the optimal treatment program for the patient.

The benefit scores can be used in a variety of ways. One is to find the best treatment for each patient. Another is to find the most effective and efficient ways to achieve a specified goal for a group of patients such as a physician's panel, members of a health plan, or employees of a corporation. Related uses are to set priorities for care management, outreach programs, or incentive programs to increase compliance.

An Archimedes team has worked with physicians and administrators in Kaiser Permanente-Hawaii to integrate this tool into KP HealthConnect. Person-specific data is extracted from KP HealthConnect on each patient every night. The Archimedes tool then calculates the risks, outcomes of treatments, and benefit scores for every patient overnight. That information is then available to physicians who will see patients the next day. The Hawaii region has developed a panel support tool (see Chapter Six) that pulls up the Archimedes-generated information and presents it to physicians and patients at the time of the patient visit. The physician and patient can then discuss the options and choose the appropriate treatment for the patient. The risks and benefit scores are also used to monitor progress and motivate the patient to continue the treatment recommendations.

In this case, the application works at the level of the individual patient, whereas in the previous example (A-L-L) the application worked at the level of a health plan or population as a whole. KP HealthConnect provides the data needed by the Archimedes tool to calculate each patient's risk and benefits of treatments. It also provides the decision support tools for passing the information to physicians and patients for their decisions. In turn, Archimedes provides the analysis and calculates the expected outcomes of different options for use by the decision makers. An evaluation of this pilot is under way to assess the optimal use of this information to improve physician and patient decision making and ultimately clinical outcomes.

Limitations of the Model

The Archimedes model was designed specifically to answer the types of questions decision makers ask, and to deliver the types of information required. However, it is important to understand the model's limitations.

The model is currently limited to the conditions and diseases listed earlier, and even within the conditions currently included, the model may not include all of the tests and treatments, especially new ones, of interest for any particular question. These limitations are being addressed by adding new conditions such as mental health disorders, osteoporosis, HIV, pregnancy, additional cancers, and so forth; and by adding any available data on new tests and treatments.

But the most important limitation pertains to its accuracy. While the validations performed to date have been very promising, they do not prove that the model will always be accurate, and in fact it has been wrong on occasion in the sense that its results have fallen outside the confidence intervals of the results of the real trial against which it was tested. In the seventy-four original validation exercises, this happened three times. Because the Archimedes model depends on current medical knowledge and evidence, it is subject to any gaps in that knowledge.

Given the model's limitations, it is important to understand the goal of the Archimedes model: it is to address the important questions at a clinically realistic level of detail and *more accurately than other available methods* for answering the questions. If it is feasible to answer a question by conducting an empirical study, then the study should be conducted. But if an empirical study is not feasible and decision makers still desire quantitative information about the consequences of the different options they face, then the goal of the Archimedes model is to provide that information as accurately as possible, given current medical science and evidence.

Of course, in the same way that medical knowledge, technology, and evidence continually improves, the Archimedes Model will continually improve. The key to improving it is access to data from formal epidemiological studies and controlled clinical trials, on one hand, and person-specific, longitudinal data, on the other, collected in the normal course of delivering health care to real populations. Fittingly, this is precisely the data that KP HealthConnect provides.

A Vision for the Future

One way to imagine what could be accomplished by linking EHRs such as KP HealthConnect to Archimedes is to think of all the different demonstration studies and clinical trials that medical scientists, in an ideal world, would conduct to answer the important questions we face in health care. We know that it is not feasible to conduct all those trials. Somehow, we have to develop other methods for answering the questions. Linking comprehensive EHRs, with vast amounts of patient data, to Archimedes is just such a method. Together, Archimedes and KP HealthConnect are capable of creating a virtual copy of the Kaiser Permanente system within the computer. That virtual world could then be used to conduct the desired studies and provide answers in the same way that Boeing experiments with various airplane designs inside of the computer, and that architects calculate how buildings will respond in earthquakes. Virtual people would get virtual diseases, develop virtual signs and symptoms, seek care from virtual providers in virtual clinics, receive tests, have diagnoses made, be admitted to hospitals, receive treatments, have outcomes, and so forth.

All of this—the population, the incidence of diseases, the care processes, the utilization, the costs—would be calibrated to match Kaiser Permanente's population and delivery system. Once built, calibrated, and validated, this virtual world could be used to answer a wide variety of questions, including forecasting the occurrence of diseases, quality, utilization, and costs into the future if nothing is changed and care continues as currently practiced. That information by itself would be invaluable for planning. But the much more powerful use of the virtual world would be to explore a variety of different options for improving quality and efficiency. That is, decision makers could use the virtual world to implement potential programs and conduct the types of clinical trials or other evaluation programs that are not feasible in reality. Because the virtual world is in a computer, decision makers could explore an almost limitless number of options that are not feasible to investigate in the "real" world.

In fact, the Archimedes Model already contains a virtual world. Currently, that world is based on national-level data from the National Health and Nutrition Evaluation Survey. Care processes are based on guidelines of national organizations; utilization is based on datasets such as the National Ambulatory Medical Care Survey and the National Hospital Discharge Survey, and costs are based on Medicare reimbursement. Because it is based on highly aggregated national-level data, the answers it produces today are generic and apply to "average" care in the United States. They are useful for general guidance, but they are not specific to any particular setting.

Creating a Virtual Kaiser Permanente World

To make the virtual world of Archimedes applicable to Kaiser Permanente it is necessary to use data from KP HealthConnect to create the virtual population, care processes, performance levels, and cost structures. In addition to providing important insights into how health care is actually delivered within the Kaiser Permanente system, and how it could be improved, such a linkage would improve the accuracy of the model's representations of physiology, disease, and care processes.

Once built, this virtual world, which we might call "Kaiser Permanente Archimedes" could then be used routinely to help design, try out, and apply the full range of clinical management tools, such as guidelines, performance measures, quality improvement projects, disease management programs, and incentive programs. It could be used to forecast utilization and costs, compare different drugs, plan new programs, compare different strategies for implementing programs, set priorities, set performance targets, and identify strategic goals. It could be used to compare performance in different regions, compare the quality of care delivered to different subpopulations, and calculate the overall score for quality and value. It would be continuously updated to track the population and care processes, to incorporate the latest research, as well as new tests and treatments, and new evidence. It would also be continuously validated by predicting new landmark clinical trials. When new programs based on the model's predictions are introduced, evaluation studies would be performed to check its accuracy, as was done with the A-L-L project described earlier.

To envision this prospect, picture the Houston Space Center, where computers are constantly monitoring the state of a rocket and capsule, its position, and its target. The trajectory of the capsule to the target has been carefully calculated, and on the basis of the feedback is constantly being adjusted. Whenever anything goes wrong, decision makers are alerted and options are instantly calculated.

Now imagine the "Kaiser Permanente Archimedes" control room, where the computer screens are displaying a wide variety of indicators of the current state of quality and efficiency of the health care system, graphs are projecting future values of the indicators, tables are comparing the effects of different strategies and programs for improving quality. Key decision makers will also have versions of the system sitting on their desks. Anyone who has a question—whether an individual physician, a department chair, a clinical committee, administrator, or a policymaker—will be able to turn to the computer and get credible quantitative answers that will enable them to understand the actual magnitudes of the different options they face. They will be able to explore a wide range of options, compare them, and choose the best way to meet their objectives.

ARCHeS: A First Step into the Future

A taste of that future can be gained by considering what might be called version 1 of the software for implementing Kaiser Permanente Archimedes. That system, called ARCHeS, is already being built with a $15.6 million grant from the Robert Wood Johnson Foundation. In just a few years, decision makers will be able to sit in front of a terminal, open a user-friendly interface, and set up their problem with the following steps:

- *Select or specify a setting.* This could be the entire health care system or a particular medical center. This will define the population, protocols, patterns of care, cost structure, and other factors that apply to their problem. They will be able to select those settings from libraries, or create new ones.
- *Specify or select a target population.* This is the specific population within the chosen setting to which they want to give interventions. An example of a target population is "all people with diabetes and either blood pressure levels above 130 or LDL levels above 100."

- *Select or specify interventions.* These are the "options" whose effects they want to explore—the particular prevention activities, tests, treatments, and other activities that will be delivered to the target population. Specifications could be as simple as "give aspirin 65 mg to everyone over forty," or could be a complex algorithm with many steps and decision points. Similarly there will be a library of existing protocols, and the ability to define new ones.
- *Select or specify outcomes.* These are the outcomes the decision makers want to measure. The choices will include biological variables and intermediate biomarkers, such as cholesterol levels or C reactive protein; clinical outcomes (heart attacks, strokes, blindness, end-stage renal disease, and so on); procedures, such as bypass operations; logistic events (office visits, admissions, and so on); medical costs (total and broken down by departments); non-medical costs (lost time from work, lost productivity); and measures of quality of life, such as life years spent with end-stage renal disease.
- *Select or specify the design.* In this step, the decision maker designates things like the number of people in the simulation, the time horizon, how the results should be reported, and the statistical methods.

These steps will be done in minutes, with none of the hassle or logistic barriers that occur in the real world. And when they finish, users of ARCHeS will press "Calculate," wait a few minutes, and then get the results. They will be able to rerun the problem as many times as they want under a variety of different assumptions and scenarios. They will be able to sort through the population to examine the results for particular groups, such as people with particular risk factors for diseases. They will be able to examine outcomes such as utilization and costs at different levels, such as pharmacy versus laboratory versus hospital admissions.

The results of the analysis will then be passed to decision makers, who will weigh in additional factors pertinent to the decision. For in the end, the decisions and choice of actions require human judgment. The contribution of ARCHeS will be to help ensure that the humans making those judgments are as well informed as possible about the consequences of the choices they face.

Conclusion

Kaiser Permanente Archimedes is made possible by two innovations: data from KP HealthConnect and the analytical powers of the Archimedes Model. Linking the two systems into one can create an entirely new system for improving the quality and efficiency of health care that will not only benefit Kaiser Permanente's members but serve as a flagship for how decisions can be made and health care can be delivered in the future.

CHAPTER TWELVE

THE DIGITAL TRANSFORMATION OF HEALTH CARE

By George C. Halvorson

Chapter Summary

This chapter examines the ongoing transition from the world of the paper-based medical record to electronic health records and the revolutionary implications of that transition for quality of care, patient-centeredness, patient safety, medical research, and the total cost of health care. It reviews how KP HealthConnect provides an early glimpse of the current and future potential for the transformation of health care delivery.

Introduction

Computers will revolutionize health care. Easy access to real-time, complete data about each patient will help physicians be better physicians.

The science of medicine is enhanced when data becomes a regular tool of both medical practice and medical research.

George C. Halvorson is the CEO and chairman of the board of Kaiser Foundation Health Plan and Kaiser Foundation Hospitals, Inc., and the author of numerous books on many aspects of health care.

Kaiser Permanente has recognized that functional reality, so it has invested billions of dollars to create a vast, real-time, fully computerized database for care delivery, and we have begun a multiyear agenda of figuring out how to use that computerized data optimally.

The rest of America should consider going down a similar path. Most health care data for America is still stored in paper medical records.

Connectivity between most American care givers in today's highly siloed world of traditional paper medical records is often so functionally difficult that far too many physicians who share patients find good patient information flow to be operationally and logistically impossible.

We are living at the tail end of the dark ages relative to medical connectivity. A decade from now, we will look back on the current lack of connectivity between patients and care givers and at the lack of connectivity between multiple care givers who serve the same patients, and we will wonder how care was actually delivered. Today's process will look as primitive to care givers ten years from now as paper-check-based banking looks to today's young people. Medical students a decade from now will not believe that it was possible to deliver good care in today's data-deprived care settings. Data will be the new stethoscope—or the new x-ray machine.

Health care has made a number of equivalent leaps forward in a number of other areas. Imagine the modern medical student who trained with only x-rays as a standard tool saying to older medical colleagues, "You mean you had to diagnose broken bones by feeling the skin over the bone with your bare fingers? You had to guess about whether a break existed? You didn't have any idea how bad a break was unless the bone stuck through the skin? That must have been horrible."

A neurology professor a couple of years ago was giving a talk, and he told about learning to figure out where in a person's brain a tumor might be by moving a lit match from side to side in front of a patient's eyes. He said he was proudly explaining how he had become fairly skilled at the technique and was telling a medical school class how to do it.

One of the students asked, "Why wouldn't you just do a scan?" He said the class looked at him holding a lit match in his hand like he was, in his words, "a witch doctor advising the use of magical chants instead of teaching them modern medicine."

Magical chants may well have their place for some health care conditions, but diagnosing the exact size and location of a brain tumor is probably done more consistently and accurately with either a CT scan or an MRI.

Unleashing the Power of Computerized Data

Computer-supported care is going to have the very same kind of "jump-shift" impact on care delivery as each of the earlier major medical breakthroughs—like discovering that germs cause disease or that antibiotics can kill germs. When the toolkit changes, medical care changes. The medical toolkit for care information is about to make a huge change. Care will never be the same, and it will be a lot better in ways we can't even anticipate.

One of our senior care leaders at Kaiser Permanente likes to say that introducing complete, real-time data to care delivery is like opening up the Internet to commerce and communications. We can't possibly anticipate all of the paths this new toolkit will take us down.

The Internet is an evolving toolkit. The Web is changing in complexity and functionality every day, in a world and a culture of continuous creativity and innovation.

Health IT will explode in the same way. In-house connectivity that is being piloted today will be perfected tomorrow. Medical research projects that historically have been set up to run for a limited period and that involve relatively few subjects in today's paper medical record data environment will be transformed into ongoing, virtually perpetual projects involving complete data on huge populations of subjects.

Both better research and better care will result.

Using Kaiser Permanente's new health record database and linking it electronically to older, historical patient data, we have recently learned that high cholesterol levels in forty-year-old men double their chance of having Alzheimer's disease in their sixties (Solomon and others, 2009). We combined old medical information in our historical files with the new Kaiser Permanente HealthConnect medical record and discovered an important correlation that no one had even suspected. When we add DNA data to our data file, we will be able to better identify exactly which people with high cholesterol are most likely to have Alzheimer's. Care will become much more personal because we will know so much more about each person.

We are just now getting access to some very powerful information—learnings that can only be acquired with longitudinal data and data about entire populations of people. Small sample sizes and truncated datasets are the number one curse of traditional medical research, and the huge expense for individually and manually collecting each piece of paper-based data is the second major curse.

Both the curse of too little data and the curse of the cost of data gathering can be eliminated by complete, longitudinal, and real-time electronic data about patients and care. You don't have to send teams of nurses physically into a paper or computer file to spend years manually sorting through individual charts to gather population data—as they did for the famous and invaluable Rand study of medical practice consistency (McGlynn and others, 2003). The Rand Study took nearly a dozen nurses working for a couple of years to do the one-time care status portrait for about 20,000 people. That is one of the best studies in the world on variability in medical practice and the use of recommended practices. That's the good news. The bad news is that the study is too expensive to update to see if anything has changed.

In the new world we are headed into, that basic study can be done electronically for much larger populations with a lot more data for a lot less money —and then updated weekly, or even hourly. The new database involves years of longitudinal tracking that can turn a research snapshot into a moving picture.

One of the next major breakthroughs in learning will definitely involve DNA. Linking DNA to an electronic medical record for a large population of people will yield golden research findings that will save lives and improve care delivery in multiple ways. Care will be much more effectively personal when our care givers have much better data about the rights, needs, chemistry, genetics, and care needs of each person.

Again, like the explosion of highly creative commercial users we see constantly emerging on the Internet, the ability of the best creative minds in health care to plumb the new data and find important linkages that no one suspected will be critically important for enabling continuous improvement for care delivery and the process of care.

Glimpses of the Tip of the Iceberg

Safety will also improve for patients when the datasets are more robust. Dangers invisible to the naked eye will be seen clearly by the electronic eye. We have already seen the tip of that iceberg.

A pre–KP HealthConnect electronic database had already raised the flag on a number of care safety issues. For instance, we were able to identify a disproportionate and totally unexpected number of Vioxx-related deaths. Kaiser Permanente pulled Vioxx out of our formulary more than six months before the rest of the country— alerted partly by our publicly announced decision—did the same (Rauber, 2004). The old Kaiser Permanente database also identified real problems over time for a number of patients with certain heart stents, resulting in new care protocols for many stent patients.

The old Kaiser Permanente database on joint replacements and joint surgeries also identified important differences in success rates for various devices and approaches to those surgeries. That research, which took advantage of the newly implemented KP HealthConnect, has also changed care practices within Kaiser Permanente, and it is changing care in the rest of the country, as well.

Moving Beyond the Data Vacuum

Computerized data and support should not be a new idea for health care. Other industries have skilled data analysts who do incredibly effective process improvement work very routinely as a matter of course in running their businesses.

Health care has never had that systematic process improvement mentality, culture, or skill set, despite the fact that there are millions of very smart people in health care. But consistent care improvement has not been on their agenda. Why is that? The lack of a continuous improvement culture in health care has been caused in part by a lack of real data about performance, outcomes, results, and care givers. No one in any industry can do continuous improvement in a data vacuum.

So the new dataset for health care will help both research and operations. It will support better and more focused day-to-day care. This is already happening. With the help of KP HealthConnect, Kaiser Permanente regions had the highest scores in the country on eight HEDIS overall quality measures in 2008. Every Kaiser Permanente region also had the highest scores in their local markets in just about all of those categories.

How did that happen? As Louise Liang pointed out in the opening chapter of this book, Kaiser Permanente did not have eight first place overall scores five years ago. Each of those "wins" was assisted by KP HealthConnect and its panel management tools and patient-focused support systems that give nurses and physicians the reminders and prompts needed to deliver highly consistent overall, continuously improving care in those care categories.

Forging a Connected World

The learning from those successful outcomes of consistent, computer-supported care should not be limited to the people and patients of Kaiser Permanente.

The entire country and the rest of the world need their own versions of KP HealthConnect. Creating "Virtual Kaiser Permanentes" should be a major policy goal for American health care. What does that mean? It means that all care givers in America need to be connectable and connected relative to the patients they share. That should be a very basic functional goal of health care reform in America. All care givers in America need to know that they have all of the needed data about each and every patient—past and current data about every test, treatment, and diagnosis for each patient.

All care givers also would be better served if all doctors had electronic connectivity with their patients. Connections happen in other areas. Patients "tweet" each other about their daily lives—and then have to communicate on paper or face-to-face with their physician. All care givers who share a patient should have connectivity with each other to provide team care to each patient. And patients should be electronically connected to their doctors and their health care information. With today's computer technology, that is entirely possible.

Virtual Kaiser Permanentes can and should be created. They can be defined, designed, developed, and then implemented with the patients as the focus of the entire health care system and the health care database. We should have a national health agenda that enables the creation of team-based, well-connected care.

The good news is that the proven and measurable success of KP HealthConnect and team care at Kaiser Permanente significantly increases the likelihood that similar systems will be created. When the world learns that the total KP HealthConnect value equation includes cutting the number of heart failures in half or cutting the number of asthma crises by a third, that learning will help people set goals. That data will give purchasers of health care a new expectation about what their patients should expect and receive from their care teams. Without those successes, care improvement in other settings is less likely to happen. There is no reason to reorganize and connect care just for philosophical or ideological reasons. But when team-care actually saves lives, the electronic connectors that enable team care will become embedded in a functioning business model in other care sites as well. The success of KP HealthConnect and its support systems is a reason for other care organizations and other health plans to follow in that path.

Realizing the Blue Sky Vision

Our own member surveys show that patients love the new electronic toolkit. In the year after secure messaging between physicians and patients was first introduced at Kaiser Permanente—supported by KP HealthConnect—one million patient contacts occurred electronically through secure messages instead of in person.

A year after that, 3.6 million such contacts happened, saving patients the time and inconvenience of having to drive to a care site to exchange basic care information with a care giver in a face-to-face encounter. In 2009, Kaiser Permanente will respond to more than six million secure e-mail messages. And new members are signing up for that and other online services every day.

Patients would now rise up in anger and rebellion if Kaiser Permanente decided to stop doing e-visits. E-connectivity works so well because with KP HealthConnect on their desktops, Kaiser Permanente care givers have at their fingertips so much data about their patients that an e-visit or telephone visit is a sensible way—even sometimes a superior way—to deliver certain kinds of care or information.

Beyond the clear convenience of e-visits and telephone visits, patients are accessing kp.org and their personal health record, My Health Manager, in record numbers for all sorts of help—information on the flu, interactive programs for weight loss, lab tests, and medication refills. Our experience suggests that these patients are more satisfied with their care, and that may ultimately lead to better health outcomes.

The Future of Computer-Supported Care

The future of health care is one of infinite possibilities, as the Blue Sky team envisioned at the start of the KP HealthConnect planning and implementation process.

Homes will increasingly become sophisticated care sites. E-visits will be blended with visual electronic connectivity tools and in-home medical monitoring devices to make a wide spectrum of care more timely, more immediate, more interactive, and much more convenient.

"Care everywhere" will continue to evolve as a care concept, and Kaiser Permanente will be just one of many organizations pioneering multiple levels of connectivity and data sharing with other health care organizations.

Three- or four-way virtual conversations, with shared medical imaging, such as X-rays, between patients, primary care doctors, and other specialists are now possible. Virtual second opinions can already be part of the normal framework of care delivery. These kinds of consults are much safer and easier to do when the care givers all share electronic health records (EHRs) with complete information on the patient's test, lab results, scans, and diagnosis.

Team care will be enhanced hugely. Real-time virtual consults with a chronic disease patient's primary care doctor, specialist, and related therapists will become standard practice—with the patient participating in the process. Kaiser Permanente is even now piloting these kinds of consults, and the early evidence suggests they work really well.

Think of the contrast. In the "old days," a doctor would say, "I think you may need a specialist for the next phase of your care. Let me write you a referral to Dr. Smith. You should call her office to set up an appointment. Here's her address. Tell her I told you to call."

The patient would then leave the care site, go home, call Dr. Smith's office, and set up an appointment with the specialist at some future time at another care site.

Too often, in the world of paper medical records, a patient seeing a new doctor brings no past or current information about his or her care or diagnosis. In the best case, the patient would carry a written referral file with paper copies of some key notes from past care sites. And the new care site would almost always start all over with all tests.

That's the old world. For people who don't get their care from electronically connected provider organizations, such as Kaiser Permanente, Mayo, Geisinger, Intermountain, Health Partners, Group Health of Puget Sound, and a very small number of team-care organizations, it's actually not the old world. It's today's world.

The new, connected world will be entirely different. In this new world, the first doctor might say, "We need an expert opinion here. Let me get Dr. Smith on our computer system and we can do a consultation right now. Dr. Smith also has your full medical record on her screen, so we don't need to send or redo any test or scan. Let's see what we can learn, together, right now, with you here in the room."

Specialty consults can now be real-time and virtual, occurring via computer in the primary care doctor's exam room—with a printout of follow-up instructions given to the patient on the spot and a secure e-message sent as a reminder and reinforcement.

Team care is possible today, and through KP HealthConnect it is happening today. Team care at Kaiser Permanente cut the death rate from both major forms of heart disease by 73 percent in our Colorado region (Sandhoff and others, 2008), and it cut the number of broken bones from osteoporosis in older patients by 37 percent in another project (Dell and others, 2008).

Making the Right Thing the Easy Thing

Connectivity is good, and team care is even better. The reason Kaiser Permanente spent nearly $4 billion putting KP HealthConnect in place is that we believe passionately in team care and we know that it takes a computer to fully connect a team. Computers can connect care givers outside of Kaiser Permanente to our care givers, as well. The two most fundamental learnings of KP HealthConnect just need to be applied to other settings that want to use computers to support care:

Learning One: Have all of the information all of the time.

Learning Two: Make the right thing easy to do.

Both of those points are actually profound lessons. They seem simple. They are, in fact, elegant. In today's world of computer connectivity, both of those strategies are possible in multiple settings if the people deciding health care policy in Washington, D.C., understand and appreciate the importance and the wisdom of each of them and set up expectations for care and connectivity accordingly.

If the right thing is hard to do, it won't get done. EHR projects in a number of other sites have failed completely because they made the right thing hard to do. That's a mistake. The right thing to do needs to be supported, not impeded, by the design of the system and process. Computers are not magical. They are tools. Tools need to be used in the context of an agenda, a strategy, and a focus on creating value.

People do not realize how much low-hanging fruit exists in American health care today. Care costs are not evenly distributed. Seventy five percent of all health care costs come from patients with chronic conditions (Centers for Disease Control and Prevention, 2009). Eighty percent of those costs come from patients with comorbidities—multiple diagnoses that involve multiple physicians (Robert Wood Johnson Foundation & Partnership for Solutions, 2004).

Our own internal data suggests that about 1 percent of patients incur about 35 percent of all costs, and 10 percent of patients incur about 80 percent of the costs. So we don't need to improve care support for most patients. But if we do a really good job on care and can keep just half of that 1 percent of high-cost patients from entering that expensive, dire-need status, we could cut the costs of total care by billions of dollars, and we could make care outcomes a lot better for Americans in the process.

We need to target better care for these patients. We need to set collective goals for care improvement—and then we need computer-based tools to help us achieve those goals.

My last book, *Health Care Will Not Reform Itself* (Halvorson, 2009), listed the ten mandates that people designing a health IT system should follow. Interestingly, those same ten points describe the characteristics of the ideal American health care database: (1) patient-focused; (2) complete; (3) accessible by all relevant parties; (4) current (real-time, if possible); (5) easy to use; (6) linked to care improvement programs; (7) accessible to patients as well as care givers; (8) transportable (when people change health plans or care givers); (9) interoperable; and (10) confidential.

Conclusion

The future of computer-supported health care is blindingly bright. We can't begin to imagine how many ways complete care data and meaningful connectivity will improve care, care delivery, and the science of care.

It is a good road to be on. KP HealthConnect was a great investment for Kaiser Permanente to make. The people inside Kaiser Permanente who put the largest non-governmental IT project in the world successfully in place deserve our great gratitude—and the people who are now very creatively using that new system and its supplementary systems to make care better are earning the gratitude of the world.

We have a lot to learn—and the learning will define us and make us better at being who we are and doing what we do.

Be well.

Appendix

Select Publications About KP HealthConnect

Chen, C., T. Garrido, D. Chock, G. Okawa, and L. Liang, "The Kaiser Permanente Electronic Health Record: Transforming and Streamlining Modalities of Care," *Health Affairs*, 2009, 28(2), 323–333.

EHRs can help achieve more-efficient contacts between patients and providers, while maintaining quality and satisfaction.

Feldstein, A., S. R. Simon, J. Schneider, M. Krall, D. Laferriere, D. H. Smith, et al., "How to Design Computerized Alerts to Ensure Safe Prescribing Practices," *Joint Commission Journal on Quality and Safety*, 2004, 30(11).

A study at Kaiser Permanente-Northwest, where prescribers have used computerized order entry since 1996, was designed to develop and evaluate medication safety alerts and processes for educating prescribers about the alerts.

Feldstein, A. C., D. H. Smith, N. Perrin, X. Yang, S. R. Simon, M. Krall, et al., "Reducing Warfarin Medication Interactions: An Interrupted Time Series Evaluation," *Archives of Internal Medicine*, 2006, 166(9), 1009–1015.

This group-randomized trial compared computerized decision support interventions to reduce the co-prescribing of warfarin and interacting medications.

Garrido, T., L. Jamieson, Y. Zhou, A. Wiesenthal, and L. Liang, "Effect of Electronic Health Records in Ambulatory Care: Retrospective, Serial Cross Sectional Study," *British Medical Journal*, 2005, 330.7491.581.

Researchers found that two years after electronic health records had been fully implemented, age-adjusted rates of office visits had fallen by 9 percent, doctors replaced some office visits with telephone contacts, and quality measure remained unchanged or slightly improved.

Garrido, T., B. Raymond, L. Jamieson, L. Liang, and A. Wiesenthal, "Making the Business Case for Hospital Information Systems—A Kaiser Permanente Investment Decision," *Journal of Health Care Finance*, 2004, 31(2), 16–25.

Further evidence in favor of the clinical IT business case is set forth in Kaiser Permanente's cost-benefit analysis for an electronic hospital information system. This article reviews the business case for an inpatient electronic medical record system, including thirty-six categories of quantifiable benefits that contribute to a positive cumulative net cash flow within an eight-and-a-half-year period.

Hsu, J., J. Huang, V. Fung, N. Robertson, H. Jimison, and R. Frankel, "Health Information Technology and Physician-Patient Interactions: Impact of Computers on Communication during Outpatient Primary Care Visits," *Journal of the American Medical Informatics Association*, 2005, 12, 474–480. DOI 10.1197/jamia.M1741.

The aim of this study was to evaluate the impact of introducing health information technology on physician-patient interactions during outpatient visits.

Hyatt, J., W. Taylor, and L. Budge, "Population Care Information Systems (PCIS): Managing the Health of Populations with KP HealthConnect," *The Permanente Journal*, Fall 2004, 8(4).

KP HealthConnect creates an opportunity to practice population care management on a scale unparalleled elsewhere on the planet. To realize this potential, the authors ask, How can KP HealthConnect support population care management in the near future and over the long term?

Okawa, G., "Integrating Evidence into KP HealthConnect: Making the Right Thing Easier to Do," *The Permanente Journal*, Spring 2005, 9(2).

Three case scenarios explore the capacity of KP HealthConnect to delivery high-quality evidence to the clinician in a form that supports and improves decision making in the exam room.

Raymond, B., "The Kaiser Permanente IT Transformation," *Healthcare Financial Management*, 2005, 59(1), 62–66.

To demonstrate and document the value of its health IT initiatives, Kaiser Permanente has developed strategies, methodologies, and models to improve the deployment and financial management of its technology investments. Eight key considerations are distilled from Kaiser Permanente's experience.

Serrato, C. A., S. Retecki, and D. E. Schmidt, "MyChart—A New Mode of Care Delivery: 2005 Personal Health Link Research Report," *The Permanente Journal*, Spring 2007, 11(2).

This study of Kaiser Permanente members found that patients were highly satisfied with the e-mail exchanges they had with their primary care provider. The study also found strong evidence that e-mail encounters reduced office visits and telephone calls to Kaiser Permanente.

Simon, S. R., D. H. Smith, A. C. Feldstein, N. Perrin, X. Yang, Y. Zhou, R. Platt, and S. B. Soumerai, "Computerized Prescribing Alerts and Group Academic Detailing to Reduce the Use of Potentially Inappropriate Medications in Older People," *Journal of the American Geriatrics Society*, 2006, 54(6), 963–968.

This five-year study adds to the evidence base supporting the use of decision support tools to reduce medication errors and improve the quality of medication prescribing in older patients.

Thompson, D., D. Classen, T. Garrido, J. Bisordi, S. Novogoratz, and W. Zywiak, "The Value of Vendor-Reported Ambulatory EHR Benefits Data," *Healthcare Financial Management*, 2007, 61(4), 82–86.

This study concludes that a benefits database maintained by an ambulatory clinical systems vendor provided information that is useful but that also has limitations.

Tong Nagy, V., and M. H. Kanter, "Implementing the Electronic Medical Record in the Exam Room: The Effect on Physician-Patient Communication and Patient Satisfaction," *The Permanente Journal*, Spring 2007, 11(2).

Patient satisfaction scores for all primary and specialty care physicians in a large medical center in Southern California did not significantly increase or decrease in the short period after computers were introduced into exam rooms.

Woods, K., M. Licht, and W. Caplan, "The Clinical Knowledge Management Process Behind KP HealthConnect," *The Permanente Journal*, Fall 2004, 8(4).

The primary focus of the clinical knowledge management process behind KP HealthConnect is the collaborative creation of rigorous, evidence-based content for clinicians to use at the point of care. The SmartTools within KP HealthConnect are key mechanisms for making that happen.

Zhou, Y. Y., T. Garrido, H. L. Chin, A. M. Wiesenthal, and L.L. Liang, "Patient Access to an Electronic Health Record with Secure Messaging: Impact on Primary Care Utilization," *American Journal of Managed Care*, 2007, 13(7), 418–424.

An evaluation of the impact of patient access to an integrated multifunction electronic personal health record that included secure patient-physician electronic messaging found statistically significant decreases in primary care office visit rates and primary care telephone contact rates.

References

Ash, J. S., Berg, M., and Coiera, E. "Some Unintended Consequences of Information Technology in Health Care: The Nature of Patient Care Information System-related Errors." *Journal of the American Medical Informatics Association*, 2004, 11, 104–112.

Bates, D. W., and others. "The Costs of Adverse Drug Events in Hospitalized Patients." *Journal of the American Medical Association*, 1997, 277, 307–311.

Bates, D. W., and others. "Effect of Computerized Physician Order Entry and a Team Intervention on Prevention of Serious Medication Errors." *Journal of the American Medical Association*, 1999, 280(15), 1311–1316.

Berwick, D., Calkins, D., McCannon, J., and Hackbarth, A. "The 100,000 Lives Campaign." *Journal of the American Medical Association*, 2006, 295(3), 324–327.

Casalino, L. P., and others. "Frequency of Failure to Inform Patients of Clinically Significant Outpatient Test Results." *Archives of Internal Medicine*, 2009, 169(12), 1123–1129.

Centers for Disease Control and Prevention. "Guidelines for the Prevention of Intravascular Catheter-related Infections." *Morbidity and Mortality Weekly Report*, 2002, 51 (No. RR-10).

Centers for Disease Control and Prevention. "An Overview of Ventilator-Associated Pneumonia." September 2005. [http://www.cdc.gov/ncidod/dhqp/dpac_ventilate.html].

Centers for Disease Control and Prevention. "Chronic Disease Control." February 2009. [http://www.cdc.gov/nccdphp/overview.htm].

Chen, C., Garrido, T., Chock, D., Okawa, G., and Liang, L. "The Kaiser Permanente Electronic Health Record: Transforming and Streamlining Modalities of Care." *Health Affairs*, 2009, 28(2), 323–333.

Christensen, C. *The Innovator's Dilemma*. Boston: Harvard Business School Press, 1997.

Classen, D. C., and others. "Development and Evaluation of the Institute for Healthcare Improvement Global Trigger Tool." *Journal of Patient Safety*, 2008, 4, 169–177.

Collins, Jim. *Good to Great*. New York: HarperCollins, 2001.

Congressional Budget Office. *Evidence on the Costs and Benefits of Health Information Technology*. Washington, D.C.: Government Printing Office, May 2008.

Cutler, D. "Will the Cost Curve Bend, Even Without Reform?" *New England Journal of Medicine*, October 8, 2009, 361(15), 1424–1425.

Dell, R., and others. "Osteoporosis Disease Management: The Role of the Orthopaedic Surgeon." *Journal of Bone and Joint Surgery* (American), 2008, 90, 188–194.

DesRoches, C. M. "Electronic Health Records in Ambulatory Care—A National Survey of Physicians." *New England Journal of Medicine*, 2008, 359(1), 50–60.

Dudl, J. R., Wang, M. C., Wong, M., and Bellows, J. "Large Scale Prevention of Myocardial Infarction and Stroke with a Simplified Bundle of Cardio-protective Medications." *American Journal of Managed Care*, 2009, 15(10), e88–e94.

Eddy, D. M., and Schlessinger, L. "Archimedes: A Trial-Validated Model of Diabetes." *Diabetes Care*, 2003a, 26, 3093–3101.

Eddy, D. M., and Schlessinger, L. "Validation of the Archimedes Diabetes Model." *Diabetes Care*, 2003b, 26, 3102–3110.

Eshleman, A. "Kaiser Permanente Online: What Is It?" *The Permanente Journal*, Winter 2001, 5(1), 75–78.

Escobar, G. J., and others. "Risk-Adjusting Hospital Inpatient Mortality Using Automated Inpatient, Outpatient, and Laboratory Databases." *Medical Care*, March, 2008, 46(3), 232–239.

Ferrara, A., Hedderson, M. H., Quesenberry, C. P., and Selby, J. V. "Prevalence of Gestational Diabetes Mellitus Detected by the National Diabetes Data Group or the Carpenter and Coustan Plasma Glucose Thresholds." *Diabetes Care*, September 2002, 9(25), 1625–1630.

Gandhi, T. K. "Fumbled Handoffs: One Dropped Ball After Another." *Annals of Internal Medicine*, March 2005, 142 (5), 352–358.

Gandhi, T. K., and others. "Missed and Delayed Diagnoses in the Ambulatory Setting: A Study of Closed Malpractice Claims." *Annals of Internal Medicine*, October 3, 2006, 145(7), 488–496.

Garrido, T., Raymond, B., Jamieson, L., Liang, L., and Wiesenthal, A. "Making the Business Case for Hospital Information Systems—A Kaiser Permanente Investment Decision." *Journal of Health Care Finance*, 2004, 31(2), 16–25.

Gonzales, R., Steiner, J. F., Lum, A., and Barrett, P. H. Jr. "Decreasing Antibiotic Use in Ambulatory Practice: Impact of a Multidimensional Intervention on the Treatment of Uncomplicated Acute Bronchitis in Adults." *Journal of the American Medical Association*, 1999, April 28, 281(16), 1512–1519.

Graham, D. J., and others. "Risk of Acute Myocardial Infarction and Sudden Cardiac Death in Patients Treated with Cyclo-oxygenase 2 Selective and Non-selective Non-Steroidal Anti-Inflammatory Drugs: Nested Case-Control Study." *Lancet*, February 5, 2005, 365(9458), 475–481.

Halvorson, G. C. *Health Care Will Not Reform Itself: A User's Guide to Refocusing and Reforming American Health Care*. New York: Productivity Press, 2009.

Hazlehurst, B., and others. "Natural Language Processing in the Electronic Medical Record: Assessing Clinician Adherence to Tobacco Treatment Guidelines." *American Journal of Preventive Medicine*, December 2005, 29(5), 434–439.

Hendrich, A., Chow, M., Skierczynski, B., and Lu, Z. "A 36-Hospital Time and Motion Study: How Do Medical-Surgical Nurses Spend Their Time?" *The Permanente Journal*, Summer 2008, 12(3), 25–34.

Hillier, T. A., and others. "Childhood Obesity and Metabolic Imprinting: the Ongoing Effects of Maternal Hyperglycemia." *Diabetes Care*, September 2007, 30(9), 2287–2292.

Institute for Healthcare Improvement. "Prevent Ventilator-Associated Pneumonia." [http://www.ihi.org/IHI/Programs/Campaign/VAP.htm.] Accessed October 2009.

Institute of Medicine. *To Err Is Human: Building a Safer Health System*. Washington, D.C.: National Academy Press, 2000.

Institute of Medicine. *Crossing the Quality Chasm: A New Health System for the 21st Century*. Washington, D.C.: National Academy Press, 2001.

Institute of Medicine. *Keeping Patients Safe: Transforming the Work Environment for Nurses*. Washington, D.C.: National Academy Press, 2004.

Jewell, K., and McGiffert, L. "To Err Is Human—To Delay Is Deadly: Ten Years Later, a Million Lives Lost, Billions of Dollars Wasted." *Consumers Union*, May 2009, 1–15.

Jha, A. K., and others. "Use of Electronic Health Records in U.S. Hospitals." *New England Journal of Medicine*, 360(16): 1628–38, April 16, 2009.

Kahn, J., Aulakh, V., and Bosworth, A. "What It Takes: Characteristics of the Ideal Personal Health Record." *Health Affairs*, 2009, 28(2), 369–376.

Kaushal, R., Shojania, K. G., and Bates, D. W. "Effects of Computerized Physician Order Entry and Clinical Decision Support Systems on Medication Safety: A Systematic Review," *Archives of Internal Medicine*, 2003, 163(12), 1409–1416.

Kurtz, S. M., and others. "Future Clinical and Economic Impact of Revision Total Hip and Knee Arthroplasty." *Journal of Bone & Joint Surgery* (American), October 2007, 89, 144–151.

The Leapfrog Group, "Leapfrog Group Hospital Survey Finds Majority of Hospitals Fail to Meet Important Quality Standards." October 2009. [http://www.leapfroggroup.org/media/file/2008_Survey_results_final_042909.pdf].

Lee, B. J., and Forbes, K. "The Role of Specialists in Managing the Health of Populations with Chronic Illness: The Example of Chronic Kidney Disease." *British Medical Journal*, 2009, 339, b2395.

McGlynn, E. A., and others. "The Quality of Health Care Delivered to Adults in the United States." *New England Journal of Medicine*, June 26, 2003, 348, 2635–2645.

Meadows, M. "Strategies to Reduce Medication Errors: How the FDA Is Working to Improve Medication Safety and What You Can Do to Help." *FDA Consumer*, May-June, 2003, 37

Moore, J. "Bad Data and PHR Adoption." Chilmark Research. April 2009. [http://chilmarkresearch.com/2009/04/13/bad-data-amp-phr-adoption/].

National Priorities Partnership. *National Priorities and Goals: Aligning Our Efforts to Transform America's Healthcare*. Washington, D.C.: National Quality Forum, 2008.

National Public Radio. "Talk of the Nation Interview with William Gibson," November 30, 1999.

Nordin, J., and others. "Influenza Vaccine Effectiveness in Preventing Hospitalizations and Deaths in Persons 65 Years or Older in Minnesota, New York, and Oregon: Data from 3 Health Plans." *Journal of Infective Disease*, 2001, 184(6), 665–670.

Paxton, E. W., Inacio, M., Slipchenko, T., and Fithian, D. C. "The Kaiser Permanente National Total Joint Replacement Registry." *The Permanente Journal*, Summer 2008, 12(3), 12–16.

Raebel, M. A., and others. "Randomized Trial to Improve Laboratory Safety Monitoring of Ongoing Drug Therapy in Ambulatory Patients. *Pharmacotherapy*, May 2006, 26(5), 619–626.

Raebel, M. A., Chester, E. A., Brand, D. W., and Magid, D. J. "Imbedding Research in Practice to Improve Medication Safety." In K. Henriksen, J. B. Battles, M. A. Keyes, and M. L. Grady, eds. *Advances in Patient Safety: New Directions and Alternative Approaches*, Vol. 4. Technology and Medication Safety. AHRQ Publication No. 08-0034-4. Rockville, MD: Agency for Healthcare Research and Quality, August 2008.

Rauber, C. "Raising Kaiser's Role, Vioxx Shines Light on Health Giant's Research." *San Francisco Business Times*, October 29, 2004.

Ries, L.A.G., and others. *SEER Cancer Statistics Review, 1975–2003*. Bethesda, MD: National Cancer Institute, 2006.

Robert Wood Johnson Foundation & Partnership for Solutions. *Chronic Conditions: Making the Case for Ongoing Care*. Update to "Chronic Care in America: A 21st Century Challenge." Partnership for Solutions and Johns Hopkins University, Baltimore, September 2004. [http://www.rwjf.org/pr/product.jsp?id=14685].

Sandhoff, B. G., Kuca, S., Rasmussen, J., and Merenich, J. A. "Collaborative Cardiac Care Service: A Multidisciplinary Approach to Caring for Patients with Coronary Artery Disease." *The Permanente Journal*, Summer 2008, 12(3), 4–11.

Schlessinger, L., and Eddy, D. M. "Archimedes: A New Model for Simulating Health Care Systems—The Mathematical Formulation." *Journal of Biomedical Informatics*, 2002, 35, 37–50.

Schmittdiel, J. A., Uratsu, C. S., Fireman, B. H., and Selby, J. V. "The Effectiveness of Diabetes Care Management in Managed Care." *American Journal of Managed Care*, May 2009, 15(5), 295–301.

Schoen, C., and others. "Primary Care and Health System Performance: Adults' Experiences in Five Countries." *Health Affairs* (Millwood), 2004 (suppl), W4–487. [PMID: 15513956].

Seniorjournal. "Medication Errors Injure 1.5 Million People, Mostly Seniors, Every Year." *Seniorjournal.com*. July 21, 2006. [http://seniorjournal.com/NEWS/Health/6-07-21-MedicationErrors.htm].

Silvestre, A., and others. "If You Build It, Will They Come? The Kaiser Permanente Model of Online Health Care." *Health Affairs*, March-April 2009, 28(2).

Smith, D. H., and others. "The Impact of Prescribing Safety Alerts for Elderly Persons in an Electronic Medical Record: An Interrupted Time Series Evaluation. *Archives of Internal Medicine*, May 22, 2006, 166(10), 1098–1104.

Solomon, A., and others. "Midlife Serum Cholesterol and Increased Risk of Alzheimer's and Vascular Dementia Three Decades Later." *Dementia and Geriatric Cognitive Disorders*, 2009, 28(1), 75–80.

Stewart, J., "KP Mid-Atlantic: Lessons Learned at Ground Zero of the Anthrax Crisis." *The Permanente Journal*, 2002, 6(1), 56–61.

Thompson, D., Classen, D., Garrido, T., Bisordi, J., Novogoratz, S., and Zywiak, W. "The Value of Vendor-Reported Ambulatory EHR Benefits Data." *Healthcare Financial Management*, 2007, 61(4), 82–86.

Thorpe, K. "Factors Accounting for the Rise in Health Care Spending in the United States: The Role of Rising Disease Prevalence and Treatment Intensity." *Public Health*, 2006, 120, 1002–1007.

Vogt, T. M., Aickin, M., Ahmed, F., and Schmidt, M. "The Prevention Index: Using Technology to Improve Quality Assessment." *Health Services Research,* June 2004, 39(3), 511–530.

Vogt, T. M., and others. "Electronic Medical Records and Prevention Quality: The Prevention Index." *American Journal of Preventive Medicine,* October 2007, 33(4), 291–296.

Wears, R. L., and Berg, M. "Computer Technology and Clinical Work—Still Waiting for Godot." *Journal of the American Medical Association,* March 9, 2005, 293(10), 1261–1263.

Wenzel, E. R., "The Impact of Hospital Acquired Blood Stream Infections." *Emerging Infectious Diseases,* March-April 2001, 7(174).

Wheelwright, S. C., and Clark, K. B. *Revolutionizing Product Development.* New York: The Free Press, 1992.

Woods, K., Licht, M., and Caplan, W. "The Clinical Knowledge Management Process Behind KP HealthConnect." *The Permanente Journal,* Fall 2004, 8(4), 57–59.

Zhou, Y. Y., Garrido, T., Chin, H. L., Wiesenthal, A. M., and Liang, L. L. "Patient Access to an Electronic Health Record with Secure Messaging: Impact on Primary Care Utilization." *American Journal of Managed Care* 2007, 13(7), 418–424. [http://www.ajmc.com/issue/managed-care/2007/2007-07-vol13-n7/Jul07-2509p418-424].

INDEX